THE NEW BOOK OF
SHIATSU

THE NEW BOOK OF
SHIATSU

VITALITY AND HEALTH THROUGH
THE ART OF TOUCH

PAUL LUNDBERG

PHOTOGRAPHY BY RUTH JENKINSON

CLASSICS

An Hachette UK Company
www.hachette.co.uk

This edition published in Great Britain in 2014 by
Gaia Books Ltd, a division of Octopus Publishing Group Ltd
Endeavour House
189 Shaftesbury Avenue
London
WC2H 8JY
www.octopusbooks.co.uk

First published in paperback in 1992 as *The Book of Shiatsu*
Revised edition published in 2004 as *The New Book of Shiatsu*
This Gaia Classics revised edition published in 2014

ISBN 978 1 85675 332 6

A CIP catalogue record for this book is available from the
British Library

Printed and bound in China

10 9 8 7 6 5 4 3 2 1

Caution
The techniques, ideas and suggestions in this book are to be
used at the reader's sole discretion and risk. Always observe
the cautions given, and consult a doctor if you are in doubt
about a medical condition.
Shiatsu is very safe when performed according to the
principles described in this book. It can be very effective in
relieving chronic discomforts as well as many minor acute
ailments and illnesses. Three medical conditions require
cautions: pregnancy, high blood pressure, epilepsy.
In pregnancy, observe the cautions on page 176 and
throughout the book. Do not apply strong pressure to the top
of the shoulders. Avoid points LI 4 (see p. 94) and Sp 6 (see p.
101), and the Yin Channels (Spleen, Kidney, and Liver) below
the knees.
For people with high blood pressure or epilepsy, do not give
shiatsu on top of the head. However, work on the limbs,
especially the legs and feet, is beneficial and safe. Avoid
leaning heavily on elderly or infirm people – especially those
with arthritis or osteoporosis (brittle bones); treat them in
the sitting position, described on pages 176–83.

CONTENTS

AUTHOR'S PREFACE

It is an honour and a privilege to be writing this preface to the third edition of *The Book of Shiatsu*. It was conceived as a basic introductory text to a subject for which I still have the greatest enthusiasm and its ongoing success reflects the warm reception and constant appreciation accorded to it, not only within the profession but especially by the wider public to whom it was equally adressed. Since the first edition appeared in 1992, it has been published in fifteen languages, remaining constantly in print in many countries. Thus it has played its part in helping establish shiatsu around the world, as a popular and versatile natural therapy and a way to personal health and self-understanding. Gratifying as this is, while the book continues to serve as a guide and a testament to shiatsu's many benefits, all thanks must be shared.

In this edition, we have sought to preserve the spirit of the original work and to further its aims by bringing a fresh eye to the design. With all new photography and illustrations as well as a fully revised text, I hope we have succeeded in improving the overall clarity and cohesion of theory and practice. I am also delighted that my friend, Paula Cox, has again contributed to this edition, with evocative new renderings of her original drawings.

Shiatsu is an evolving therapeutic practice with many possible applications and levels of use. It belongs to the modern world just as much as to the hardy and venerable tradition of East Asian medicine that began in China over two and a half thousand years ago. Although barely half a century has passed since modern Shiatsu was officially approved in Japan, it soon spread to the West and has grown steadily to become a globally recognized treatment method. Yet many people might still ask, "What is it that distinguishes shiatsu among the numerous forms of manual therapy today?" And in order to ensure that shiatsu's valuable contribution to our general health and wellbeing continues, we must always be prepared to answer. I suggest there might be three parts to a complete response:

1) Shiatsu is, in theory and practice, understandable, coherent and logical. It incorporates modern anatomy and physiology and does not depend on mystifying symbols

and obscure techniques. The medical tradition of China and Japan represents centuries of continual investigation and experience based on an integrated, holistic view of human beings and their environment. In that view, nature, body and mind were not separated and the universal, dynamic principles of subtle energy were appreciated long before their discovery by modern science.

2) Shiatsu is down to earth, immediately accessible and practical in application. It can be practised and enjoyed in simple form, for oneself or for others, by anyone with an interest. Thus it is valuable for personal health and wellbeing, first-aid and care in the family and community.

3) Its finely graded techniques range from the most basic to the most refined. With correct training and patience, shiatsu becomes a powerful healing method. Subtle perceptions and skills grow alongside sensitivity, autonomy, confidence and compassion in response to our shared human condition.

Shiatsu clearly offers a range of valuable options for contemporary society. When studied and practised as a skilled professional therapy, integrating traditional and modern medical knowledge, it can confidently take its place among today's most effective treatment methods and health support systems. Beyond this it has an important educational role promoting health and wellbeing in the wider community. Its most basic principles can be learned in a few weeks by anyone and practised safely at home. Shiatsu also offers natural and easy access to many systems of exercise for maintaining fitness and health.

To this adaptability throughout the intermediate range of healthcare needs must be added the glaring economic benefits of all manual therapies and healing methods. As learned, they are an internally held cultural resource, essentially free of material costs.

In offering these many benefits to contemporary society, shiatsu also conforms with the highest ideal of Eastern Traditional Medicine, ultimately guiding people towards understanding and responsibility for their own health and happiness. I hope that you enjoy your own shiatsu journey.

INTRODUCTION

Shiatsu is a Japanese word meaning "finger pressure". It is a new name, coined in the early 20th century, for the oldest form of medicine – healing with hands. Everybody has the healing power of touch and responds to touch. It is a natural ability that people are now beginning to recognize again. Shiatsu uses hand pressure and manipulative techniques to adjust the body's physical structure and its natural inner energies, to help ward off illness, and maintain good health.

Shiatsu is characterized by its great simplicity. It grew from earlier forms of massage, called Anma in Japan (Anmo or Tuina in China) which use rubbing, stroking, squeezing, tapping, pushing, and pulling to influence the muscles and circulatory systems of the body. Shiatsu, by contrast, uses few techniques and to an observer it would appear that little is happening – merely a still, relaxed pressure at various points on the body with the hand or thumb, an easy leaning of the elbows or a simple rotation of a limb. It almost seems a lazy activity and, to the extent that it conserves one's energy, it is. But underneath the uncomplicated movements much is happening internally to the body's energy on a subtle level.

Subtle energy in the body

The Eastern tradition has long described the world in terms of energy. All things are considered to be manifestsations of a vital universal force, called "Ki" by the Japanese, and "Chi", or "Qi", in China. Because of the Japanese origins of shiatsu therapy, the Japanese word Ki is used in preference to the Chinese word, Qi. Ki is the primary substance and motive force of life. It is most often described as "energy", but Ki is also synonymous with breath in the Japanese and Chinese languages. In Oriental medicine, harmony of Ki within the human body is conceived as being essential to health. All its endeavours are addressed to this end.

The aims of this book

This book is written for both "givers" and "receivers" of shiatsu. Shiatsu is for sharing with others, and you can enhance your health and your enjoyment of life by following the demonstrations illustrated in the book. By learning the basic principles of traditional Oriental medicine, you can also use your shiatsu to help when your friends or members of your family are unwell.

The study of the treatment of disease, or individual symptoms, can lead to a limited view of shiatsu and its benefits. So this book gives you a grounding in techniques and pathways for working on the body, from which you can develop your understanding of the body's "energetic" systems – the self-regulating network of subtle forces that is the basis of our health and vitality. Rather than concentrating on curing diseases, you will gain a feeling for the relationship between illness and health. Shiatsu can help you to even out the swings between extremes, find an appropriate balance, and live more fully and creatively.

The development of shiatsu in Japan

Shiatsu was developed in the early part of the 20th century by a Japanese practitioner, Tamai Tempeki, who incorporated the newer Western medical knowledge of anatomy and physiology into several older methods of treatment. Originally he called it "Shiatsu Ryoho", or "finger pressure way of healing", then "Shiatsu Ho", "finger pressure method". Now known simply as "shiatsu", it was officially recognized as a therapy by the Japanese Government in 1964, so distinguishing it from the older form of traditional massage, Anma. The role of trained shiatsu therapists is to diagnose and treat according to the principles of traditional Oriental medicine, but Tempeki also emphasized the natural principles of healing that lie behind the theory. We can access these through the simplest forms of shiatsu touch, even as beginners.

Chinese origins of shiatsu

The earliest known book of Chinese medicine is called the *Huang Ti Nei Ching* (*The Yellow Emperor's Classic of Internal Medicine*). In it the legendary Emperor questions his physician, Ch'i Po, about problems of medicine and health among his people. In one well-known passage Ch'i Po explains that different forms of medicine were developed in different regions according to the prevailing climate and the resulting constitutional problems from which people suffered. Treatment using herbs, needles, and heat were attributed to Northern, Southern, Eastern, and Western regions, but development of physical therapy including massage and breathing exercise was accorded to the people of China's central region. Thus began the long association of massage and manipulative therapy with special physical exercise, breathing techniques, and healing meditations which represented the highest level of Chinese medicine. These came to be known collectively as "Daoyin", methods for guiding the subtle energies within the body to flow smoothly. In turn, these became "Do-in" in Japan and Shiatsu is the modern inheritor of this tradition. Chinese medicine was introduced to Japan by Buddhist monks in the 6th century, but the Japanese developed and refined many of its methods to suit their own physiology, temperament, and climate. In particular they developed the manual healing and diagnostic arts, evolving special techniques of abdominal diagnosis, treatment, and abdominal massage (see pp. 162–63).

Styles of shiatsu

Many early shiatsu practitioners developed their own style and some, including Tokojiro Namikoshi and Shizuto Masunaga, founded schools that helped establish shiatsu as a therapy. There are many different styles of shiatsu today. Some concentrate on "acupressure points" (named after acupuncture), some emphasize a more formal pattern of work around the body and some follow the traditional meridians or formally recognized pathways of "Ki". Some schools highlight different diagnostic approaches, such as the "Five Element" system or Yin and Yang and the differentiation of "meridian functions". All of these are based in Eastern traditional medicine. This book is intended as a broadly based guide to shiatsu, drawing on the most useful and practical aspects of the different approaches, with Japanese "Hara Diagnosis" and sensitive bodywork at the core and the basic theories of traditional medicine as a guide. Still, the "Zen Shiatsu" of Shizuto Masunaga warrants a special mention.

Zen Shiatsu

Shizuto Masunaga incorporated his studies of both Western psychology and Chinese medicine into his experience of shiatsu; he also refined the existing methods of diagnosis. His system incorporated a new description of the pathways of Ki (Extended Meridians), special exercises known as "Makko Ho" to stimulate the flow of Ki, and a set of guiding principles to make shiatsu techniques more effective. He called his system "Zen Shiatsu" after the simple and direct approach to spirituality of the Zen Buddhist monks in Japan. This book introduces some valuable aspects of Masunaga's approach – the first principles of touch, the meridian "expressions" and related exercises. However, it shows only the classical meridians, including their internal paths, with their time-honoured links and groupings. This is all you need for good shiatsu and a sound traditional basis for further studies in formal Zen Shiatsu, or any other style.

The Eastern approach to the body and health

In this book, you may notice a circularity in the logic of East-Asian medicine. Westerners think of cause and effect as a linear progression of ideas and events from A, through B, to C. Eastern philosopy regards events as mutually conditioned, arising together. They are not seen as distinct from the environment in which they occur. The background is as important as the foreground. An example is given here to help to clarify the difference.

A headache is not just an event in the head, according to the traditional view, nor is it merely a pain, or something to be stopped without regard for its origins, nor even treated on the same basis as someone else's headache. Rather, it is an obstruction of Ki, related to the overall energy patterns in the whole body of the particular individual, their circumstances, and lifestyle. Treatment might involve work on the arms or legs as well as (or instead of) the head and will bring more lasting and satisfactory changes than will an attempt to block the superficial symptoms with a drug. Observe the cautions given on page 4.

Japanese or Chinese?

Shiatsu is Japanese by tradition and in character. However, Chinese medicine has had a constantly recurring influence in Japan, from its early introduction through to the modern era. In the second half of the 20th century, the Chinese undertook a complete revision of traditional medicine, attempting to conserve the most effective treatment methods. This has aided the understanding and influenced the evolution of contemporary shiatsu worldwide.

HOW TO USE THIS BOOK

The Book of Shiatsu is a comprehensive introduction to the use of gentle manipulation and hand pressure to bring health and vitality to your life. It is for the interested novice as well as the shiatsu student; for givers and receivers of shiatsu alike. Part One illustrates and describes in detail the fundamentals of Oriental Medicine, prepares you physically and mentally for beginning shiatsu, and explains the techniques to use and the principles to follow. It ends with a simple shiatsu routine.

Part Two presents three more detailed routines, which, together, cover all the pathways of your work on the body. The chapters in Part Two describe in detail the functions of each of the vital organs, as well as the symptoms associated with them.

Part Three extends your knowledge into the area of traditional diagnosis, and encourages you to adapt your work to suit the particular needs of your shiatsu partner.

Initial capital letters on some anatomical words indicate their Oriental meaning, which has wider connotations than the same words in the West.

A note on clothing

A shiatsu session can take place with both participants comfortably dressed in loose clothing. No special clothing is necessary.

It is important to observe the cautions given on page 4.

1. THE ORIENTAL TRADITION

The traditional Oriental view of health takes wholeness as its starting point. It recognizes the universe as an energy field and all it contains as manifestations of energy in different patterns. Though infinitely varied, everything in the universe is connected; people are an intimate part of their environment and depend on it as much as they influence it. The primary tenet of Oriental medicine is to live in accord with nature, rather than trying to adapt nature to the needs of people.

Oriental medicine is based on observation of people and their response to the environment over thousands of years. Without the anatomical knowledge made available much later, Oriental theory established its own framework to explain how the body works and to explain natural phenomena (see Yin and Yang, pp. 14–19). The focus of attention is on how to maintain harmony within the body and with the outside world.

The Chinese observed the influence of the natural world and linked people's tendencies to particular types of ailment to the characteristics of the natural world (see The Five Elements, pp. 20–23). The emotions and lifestyle were also acknowledged as contributory factors in health and disease. To stay healthy, a person must continually adapt to the changes going on, both inside the body and out. If these adaptations are not made, illness manifests as disharmony within the body. Universal energy, called Ki, flows within the body forming a matrix that links the vital Organs with all the other parts. In treatment the emphasis is on restoring harmony to the Ki in the body. The physician's task is twofold: to interpret the cause, then to advise on appropriate lifestyle adjustments and to find a means of restoring the functions of the body.

YIN AND YANG

The 8 trigrams of the I Ching

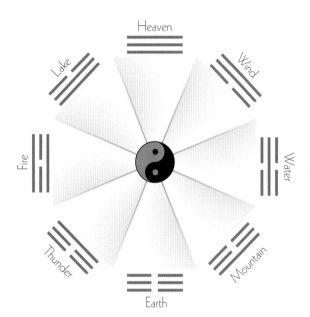

Heaven

Wind

Lake

Water

Fire

Thunder

Mountain

Earth

Yin and Yang are concepts that are central to the unique viewpoint of traditional philosophy, science, and culture in China and Japan. Established from the observation of nature and society, they came to form the basis of traditional Chinese medicine, which then spread to Japan. Understanding the role of Yin and Yang is essential in learning about shiatsu: it forms the basis for all diagnosis and treatment.

Yin–Yang theory was first elaborated in the ancient and famous Chinese book of divination, *The Book of Changes* (*I Ching*), which dates in its earliest form to the 2nd millennium BC. It was well established

Yin

Yang

陽

The Chinese characters for Yin and Yang mean, literally, the shady side and the sunny side of a hill, respectively. The hill represents existence, the "ground" in and around which Yin and Yang are in constant but ever-changing interplay. Alone, Yin and Yang have no meaning. They cannot be separated either from each other or from existence itself.

The Tao

According to Lao Tzu (6th century BC), everything in the universe arose from the "Great Ultimate Source", or Tai Chi, represented by the famous symbol . Beyond this was only emptiness, Wu Chi, represented as an empty circle ◯. The light and dark segments indicate the inherent duality in all things, as well as the interaction of Yin and Yang — the dynamic out of which life and all phenomena arise and continue to move and change. The law governing all these transformations was called the "Tao", meaning the "Way" of nature.

Yin and Yang in Nature

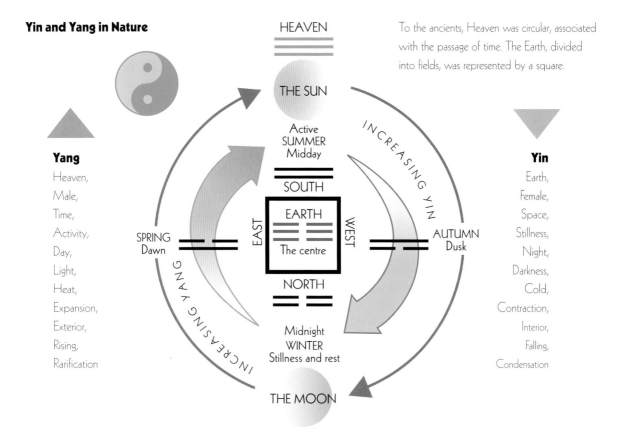

HEAVEN

To the ancients, Heaven was circular, associated with the passage of time. The Earth, divided into fields, was represented by a square.

THE SUN

Yang

Heaven,
Male,
Time,
Activity,
Day,
Light,
Heat,
Expansion,
Exterior,
Rising,
Rarification

Active
SUMMER
Midday

SOUTH

EARTH

The centre

EAST

WEST

SPRING
Dawn

AUTUMN
Dusk

NORTH

Midnight
WINTER
Stillness and rest

INCREASING YIN

INCREASING YANG

THE MOON

Yin

Earth,
Female,
Space,
Stillness,
Night,
Darkness,
Cold,
Contraction,
Interior,
Falling,
Condensation

by the time of Confucius, who added his commentaries in the 5th century BC. In this book Yang was represented by a continuous or "firm" line ———— conveying direction and movement, and Yin by a broken or "yielding" line —— —— suggesting space and stillness. These lines were grouped in eight combinations of three, symbolizing all the basic permutations of natural forces and phenomena. Among these, three Yang lines grouped together ☰ represented "Heaven", the Yang archetype of the creative, active principle. Three Yin lines ☷ represented "Earth", the receptive or passive

principle. Yang was regarded as masculine and Yin as feminine, and all life was seen as being dependent on their harmonious interaction. Light, warmth, and the passage of time were associated with the sun and its movement through Heaven; Earth offered material nourishment – food from the fields, shelter, and rest. The changing seasons and the repeating cycle of nights and days were deemed to be natural indications of the interrelatedness of Yin and Yang.

Unlike the idea of opposites inherited by Western culture from early Greek philosophy, the opposing qualities of Yin and Yang are seen as complementary and interdependent. They both create and control each other. When Yin declines, Yang expands, and vice versa, but there are no absolutes. Nothing can be wholly Yin or wholly Yang. Each contains the seed of the other: Yang will change into Yin; Yin into Yang.

Because everything has Yin and Yang characteristics to varying degrees, things can only be Yin or Yang relative to each other. Relative to the sun, the moon is Yin (cold, dense), but even the pale and watery moonlight is Yang relative to the surrounding night, and the shadowy caves and hollows where no light reaches.

Ki

The Oriental view of life, nature, and the body is firmly founded on the notion of a vital force, or energy, which can be compared with the prana of Indian yogic philosophy. Its significance is so great in Oriental thinking, and its meaning so full of breadth and subtlety, that it is best to use the untranslated word "Ki" in the same way as we have become accustomed to use the Chinese words Yin and Yang.

Energy and matter

Ki arises from the interaction of Yin and Yang, and is the primary substance of the universe. This profoundly elegant understanding has existed in Eastern cultures for thousands of years. So it is said that all things are formed from Ki and that every different thing is determined or characterized by its Ki. Ki encompasses both the material and the non-material. In its "purer" form it is subtle and rarefied; it is "substance

with no form". It is more Yang. Matter, on the other hand, is a condensed, "slowed-down" form of Ki. This is more Yin. It may seem paradoxical that Ki should exist as both matter and non-matter, but you may understand it more easily in terms of transformation and change.

Take the simple example of water boiling in a pot, transforming into steam, then condensing into droplets. Water is a more Yin state, steam is more Yang. The heat of the fire needed to boil water is intensely Yang (active), transforming the water into an expanded, Yang form. Coldness – relatively Yin – causes the condensation to form droplets that collect on cooler surfaces or fall to earth. The most Yin form of water is ice. Ki is manifest in both the transformation and the substance: Yin Ki (of water) transforming into Yang Ki (steam) and then back into water. The paradox is contained. Ki is both matter and its capacity to change. The universe, in its state of flux, sees the constant interplay of Yin and Yang, matter and non-matter.

Human Being results from the Ki of Heaven and Earth. The union of the Ki of Heaven and Earth is called Human Being.
  The Yellow Emperor's Classic of Internal Medicine (c. 100 BC)

When Ki condenses it can form Beings.
  Quote attributed to Zhu Xi (12th century AD)

Yin and Yang related to the body – structure, posture, and use

The living body has shape, structure, and weight. These are its Yin qualities. It is also active, warm, and responsive to its environment – attributes that are essentially Yang.

The head and the upper part of the body are more Yang; they are nearer Heaven. The feet and lower parts are more Yin; they are closer to the Earth.

The back and the exposed surfaces of the limbs are Yang. When we turn our backs against a cold wind, these are the strong, protective aspects we present to the outside.

The front and the protected inner aspects of the limbs are Yin. When we curl up in a defensive "armadillo" position, these are the soft, vulnerable inner surfaces that we seek to protect.

The skin, the outermost layer of the physical body, and the muscles, the active body tissue that enables us to move, are both Yang.

The bones, the deepest, hardest, and most stable of the structural tissues, are Yin. So also are the internal organs, protected within the ribcage and the pelvic cavity. These are the deepest, most essential layer of our being.

Yin and Yang in the body
Within the body, Yin and Yang influences are always at work. The roles of Yin and Yang within the body structure are summarized above.

Yin, Yang, and Ki in the body

The body depends on Ki, Blood and other essential substances, which change, flow, and circulate, and so are more Yang than the structural elements of the body. But here, too, Yin and Yang are at play together. Within the body Ki circulates in Channels, often called Meridians, which have no material form. Ki, similarly, has no physical structure and is,

therefore, relatively Yang. It is the transforming power of the inner organs and is associated with activity, protection, and warmth. Traditionally, Ki is subdivided into many types according to its role in the body.

Blood is a liquid or materialized form of Ki. Its qualities are accordingly relatively Yin. Blood nourishes and supports the physical growth and renewal of body tissues and organs. It circulates in the blood vessels and has a close relationship with the Body Fluids.

Ki and Blood support and complement each other. The Blood needs the Ki to keep it moving. The Ki needs the Blood to nourish the organs that generate it. Some Ki therefore flows with the Blood in the vessels and there is some Blood with the Ki in the Channels. "Ki is the leader of Blood; Blood is the mother of Ki." (*The Yellow Emperor's Classic of Internal Medicine*, c. 100 BC)

Body Fluids

Body Fluids are the most Yin of the body substances. This general category includes the thick (most Yin) fluids that nourish the spinal cord and brain, and the thin (more Yang) lubricating fluids, including saliva, sweat, and tears, that moisten the skin and lubricate the openings of the sensory organs. The Body Fluids also include the Blood and have nourishing, soothing, and cooling properties.

Mind and the spiritual attributes

The Chinese conceived the Spirit, or Mind, as a very rarefied body substance, the most Yang of all, associated with consciousness, intelligence, and will. The various aspects of the Spirit were thought to be housed in the Yin organs (see p. 21).

Organs, Channels, and the direction of Ki

Not only does Yin–Yang theory explain the relationship between the internal organs of the body, it also describes an "energetic" relationship between its inner and outer aspects – the vital organs and the surface. The supreme achievement of traditional Chinese medicine was perhaps that it perceived the inner organs as centres of transformation and distribution, which literally "organized" the entire body. This "organization" is mediated by the system of Channels that carries the Ki to all parts. It flows from within and circulates near the surface of the body. The internal condition of the body is reflected on the outside; work on the outside can affect the inside. In health, this is the body's regulating mechanism and allows us to adjust to the environment. In sickness, the mechanism breaks down, symptoms are produced on the outside. The ability to move Ki inside the body by giving treatment from the outside arises from the continuity of the energy network between inside and out. This is the "energetic" relationship.

The 12 main, or "Primary" Channels (see pp. 70–77) are dominated by the influence of either Heaven or Earth, producing accordingly either a downward flow from Heaven (Yang) or an upward flow from Earth (Yin). The Yang Channels are found on the back and on the outside surfaces of the arms and legs. They belong to the more superficial or "hollow" Organs of the digestive tract, principally the Stomach, Large and Small Intestines, Bladder, and Gall Bladder. Yang Organs are concerned with the processing of food and the elimination of waste; they are involved in the body's defensive functions and they are often implicated in the early or acute stages of illness. The Yin Channels are located on the front of the body and the inner surfaces of the limbs. They belong to the deep, "solid" Organs – the Lungs, Spleen, Heart, Kidneys, and Liver. The role of the Yin Organs is the transformation, storage, and distribution of Ki and Blood and they are most affected in longstanding illness or weakness. The Yin and Yang Organs complement each other: each Yin Organ is paired with a Yang Organ in a reciprocal relationship (see pp. 76–7).

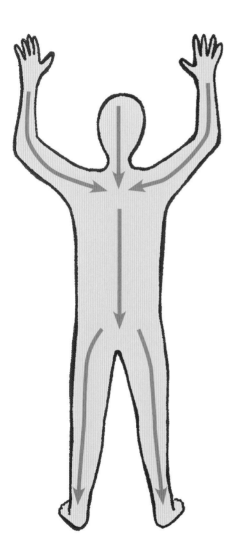

The Yang Channels flow downward, on the backs of the arms and legs.

The Yin Channels flow up the front, inner surfaces of the body.

THE FIVE ELEMENTS

The theory of Yin and Yang was not the only way by which the ancient Chinese interpreted the world. Early in the 1st millennium BC another system began to emerge in which all phenomena were seen as manifesting through one of five primary modes of Ki. These were known as the Five Elements, Five Transformations, or Five Phases, and were symbolically described as Water, Fire, Wood, Metal, and Earth. The *Shang Shu*, a text from this period, describes their qualities:

"That which soaks and descends (Water) is salty, that which blazes upwards (Fire) is bitter, that which can be bent and straightened (Wood) is sour, that which can be moulded and become hard (Metal) is pungent, that which permits sowing and reaping (Earth) is sweet."

The Five Elements were especially associated with the seasons, but also with colours, sounds, mythical animals, grains, and many other things and events. So a system of correspondences gradually developed to build up a picture of the connections in the natural world (see the chart opposite).

Around the 4th century BC, a time of turmoil and change in China, the search for order and meaning in the relationship between people and their environment led to the expansion of the Five Element theory. Things were more than just categorized; their capacity to change, interact, and transform into each other was recognized and described in various ways.

The early physicians based their understanding of the cause and development of illness on the interrelating patterns of the Five Elements (see p. 22). Each Organ was either nourished or controlled by one of the others. Disease could progress from one Organ to another through lack of nourishment, "over-control", or its opposite, "insult". Treatment of a deficient

When the Emperor Huang Ti questioned his physician Ch'i Po, he answered: "The East creates the wind; wind creates the wood; wood creates the sour flavour. The sour flavour strengthens the Liver, the Liver nourishes the tendons, the tendons strengthen the Heart and the Liver governs the eyes. The eyes see the darkness and mystery of Heaven and they discover the Tao, the Right Way among Mankind.

Anger is injurious to the Liver, but pensiveness counteracts anger. Wind is injurious to the tendons but heat and dryness counteract the wind. The sour flavour can injure the tendons but the pungent flavour counteracts the sour flavour."

The Yellow Emperor's Classic of Internal Medicine (c. 100 BC)

The Five Elements

NATURE	Wood	Fire	Earth	Metal	Water
Directions	East	South	Centre	West	North
Seasons	Spring	Summer	Transition	Autumn	Winter
Climates	Wind	Heat	Dampness	Dryness	Cold
Cyclic Stages	Birth	Growth	Ripening	Harvest	Storing
Colours	Green	Red	Yellow	White	Black/Blue
Flavours	Sour	Bitter	Sweet	Pungent	Salty

HUMAN BODY	Wood	Fire	Earth	Metal	Water
Yin Organs	Liver	Heart	Spleen	Lungs	Kidneys
Yang Organs	Gall Bladder	Small Intestine	Stomach	Large Intestine	Bladder
Sense Organs	Eyes	Tongue	Mouth	Nose	Ears
Senses	Sight	Speech	Taste	Smell	Hearing
Body Tissues	Ligaments and Tendons	Blood Vessels	Muscles (flesh)	Skin	Bones
Manifestation	Nails	Face (complexion)	Lips	Body Hair	Head Hair
Fluids	Tears	Sweat	Saliva	Mucus	Urine
Sounds	Shouting	Laughing	Singing	Weeping	Groaning
Emotions	Anger	Joy	Pensiveness/Worry	Grief	Fear
Spiritual Aspects	Ethereal Soul	Mind	Intellect	Corporeal Soul	Will

Development of the Five-Element theory

The Five Elements soon became integrated into Yin–Yang theory and the two were developed together by a philosophical school called the Naturalists. An early model of the Five Element relationships is reminiscent of the Yin–Yang diagram (see right and p. 15). This early model shows the important balance between Water and Fire, with Water representing downward movement, stillness, and rest, but full of potential power; and Fire representing upward movement and climax of activity. The complementary yet opposing tendencies, Wood and Metal, representing expansion or outward movement and contraction or inward movement respectively. Earth was seen as a moderating influence on the season, having no season of its own. It is like a pivot or reference point for change.

Later, other arrangements were developed in which Earth occupied a position equal to the other Elements — two in particular became established for representing natural order in the world; both the way in which things progress and support each other, called the generating sequence (see right), and the way in which they restrain or limit each other, called the controlling sequence (see far right).

Early Yin–Yang model representing the Five Elements

Generating sequence

Wood fuels Fire; Fire's ashes enrich the Earth; Metal is found in the Earth; Water condenses on Metal; and Water in turn feeds Wood.

Controlling sequence

Wood (plant matter) stabilizes the Earth; Earth contains Water within its banks; Water controls Fire; Fire melts Metal; and Metal (tools) cuts Wood.

or malfunctioning Organ was often given by strengthening the Organ preceding it in the sequence known as the "generating sequence" (see opposite).

The usefulness of this system extends beyond the portrayal of harmonious interaction since it can also predict or interpret the effects of disharmony, when things get "out of phase" and inevitably balance is lost. For example, if Fire is weak the effect of Water will be more than mere control, threatening to extinguish it altogether. This is known as over-acting of one Element on another. Similarly, if Water is deficient then Fire can vaporize it, thus overcoming the Element that usually controls it. This reversal of the controlling sequence is called counteracting, or "insulting".

The development of medicine progressed with the extension of the Five Element theory to include the body's major Organs, the sensory Organs and body tissues, the human emotions, and subtle spiritual qualities. Combined with external factors, such as season, climate, foods, and so on (see pp. 147–49), the whole picture of correspondences provided a reference for diagnosis and healing. A table of the traditional Five Element correspondences is given above.

As Chinese medicine developed through the centuries, the Five Elements were accorded greater or lesser importance, but their usefulness is still widely recognized today as a general system of medical reference. The Five Element system is particularly well regarded in Japan and the practice of shiatsu is greatly enhanced by a knowledge of this traditional approach.

2. YOUR OWN WELLBEING

To heal others, begin with yourself. Giving shiatsu to your friends will not be easy if you are tired, frustrated, weak, or sick. Whatever your constitution, good health springs from maintaining a balance in your diet, exercise, rest, security, level of challenge, and so on. Finding this balance means looking after yourself physically, mentally, and emotionally, and taking responsibility for your own condition. This may not be easy: self-discovery is a lifetime's work. Acknowledge your weaknesses as well as your strengths; learn to recognize when you need help and ask for it; accept as well as give.

All these are important steps on the way to gaining an inner harmony that will bring healing qualities to your work.

Shiatsu helps you on this path. As a way to health it is as enjoyable to give as to receive, and the practice of shiatsu develops not only your physical fitness but your intuition and understanding as well. This chapter presents traditional healing exercises for the practitioner and receiver, which integrate Body, Breath, and Mind, and harmonize Yin and Yang. You will gain these subtle internal benefits through grounding exercises (see pp. 26–33), breathing exercises (see pp. 36–39), and sometimes through the use of visualization or concentration. Such exercises are central to the practice of shiatsu, for beginners as well as the more accomplished.

Most shiatsu sessions take place on the floor. The grounding exercises at the beginning of this chapter are designed to give you a "feel" for the ground and to develop the flexibility and strength to enable you to work at floor level for extended periods. Exercises to allow you to obtain the same level of flexibility and strength in your fingers, your basic tools in shiatsu, are shown on pp. 34–35.

GROUNDING

To practise shiatsu well, you must learn what it means to be in touch with the ground and feel its effect on the physical body. Gravity, the "Earth-Force", conditions our total experience. From infancy we have to contend with it. Our muscular system is engaged from the outset in the effort of raising up the head, wriggling, crawling, and eventually learning to stand and walk. This process develops the secondary curves of the spine – in the neck and lumbar region – and influences our posture, grace, and balance from an early age.

Begin with some exercises on the floor to enhance your connection with the ground and remove the tensions produced by standing upright (see pp. 30–33). The exercises on all fours (see pp. 28–29) will loosen and balance the curves of your spine and benefit your nervous system. Grounding exercises increase your awareness of your body weight. They will teach you to use the ground for support: to get down and make friends with the floor; to crawl, kneel, or squat, and move comfortably on all fours. We need to feel and imbue our bodies with this feeling of support in order to convey it in our work with others.

Practice time

Create your own routine from the exercises described on the following pages. Do the exercises at any convenient time, not necessarily before giving shiatsu. You need only practise for 10–30 minutes at a time, but as your stamina improves you may want to work for longer. Practise every day if you want to, but three or four times a week is still useful. Your body will tell you what your needs and limitations are if you listen.

Comfort and safety

When giving shiatsu or practising the preparatory exercises that follow you should wear loose, comfortable clothes to allow full freedom of movement. Garments made from natural fibres help prevent overheating. Put on a sweater after exercising to prevent you from getting chilled. Avoid draughts.

Be sensible about these exercises. Don't push or strain. Work into any stiffness and resistance gradually. Look after yourself. The exercises are designed to enhance your power as a healer.

BOWING

Bowing is used both as a social and religious gesture among Eastern peoples. It signifies respect and service to another person or "higher being". In Japan the practice of bowing has many nuances, which help to smooth the passage of daily life. It is also an essential part of martial arts practice for students, teachers, and opponents.

Bowing is not only symbolic. As with many rituals, there is a practical purpose to it. It has a very calming, purifying, and focusing effect on the body and mind and makes an appropriate starting point for your exercises on the floor. Sometimes there is space for a bow between giver and receiver of Shiatsu.

1. Kneel comfortably on the floor, or on a cushion. Bring your palms together at chest level, arms slightly extended. Relax, exhale, and then inhaling deeply, imagine "Heaven's Energy" flowing down through your hands or the top of your head as you fill your lungs.

2. Exhale easily and slowly, dipping your head a little while opening your hands in symbolic offering to the "Heaven Force". Inhale and return to the starting position.

3. Now exhale deeply and fold forward at the hips. Separate your hands to place them, palms down, on the floor. Relax completely, chest on knees. Let your forehead touch the ground or "Earth". Remain quiet and still, momentarily giving up all your thoughts. Allow your next inhalation to fill your body and, thinking of life breathing into you, return naturally to the upright position.

ON ALL FOURS

This series of exercises, based on the "dog postures" of yoga, will help to counteract any stiffness in your spine by first stretching it, then relaxing it. It allows you to feel the physical weight of your chest and belly, which should literally hang from your spine, supported at each end by your arms and legs. Each exercise begins from a comfortable "all fours" position with your arms and thighs at right angles to the ground.

1. Relax on all fours. Now let your head drop and, inhaling, arch your spine high.

2. Stretch your back in the arched position, pause, then on a long, easy out breath let your back relax right down, so your spine hangs naturally. Breathe easily for a few moments and repeat.

3. Start in the "all fours" position. Tuck in your toes, then lift yourself off your knees, stretch your legs back, and raise your buttocks toward the sky. Press back from your hands, relaxing your head, and let your chest move toward your legs to narrow the inverted "V" shape. Stretch your knees and lower your heels. They need not touch the floor. Exhale as you move into and out of this position. Breathe easily as you hold it for a few moments.

4. Exhale and lower your hips to the floor, supporting the front of your body on your hands. Now raise and tighten your knees, stretching your legs, toes flat. Look up to the sky, but don't strain your head back. Breathe easily, holding the position for just a few moments.

5. Finally, relax by sinking on to your haunches, folding at the hips. Let your chest rest on your thighs, and your head touch the ground. Place your arms forward, as shown here, or alongside your legs. Breathe into your belly. This "pose of the child" is rejuvenating and relaxing.

Shifting the weight

This exercise develops a fluidity of movement between hips, spine, and shoulder joints, and strength and flexibility in the wrists. It also familiarizes you with the feeling of shifting your centre of gravity to transfer weight through your limbs in your shiatsu sessions.

Still on all fours, relax your spine and belly and begin slow, clockwise movements. Bring your body weight forward on to your left, then right hand, then back into your right and left hips. Make several circles, then reverse the direction.

Belly consciousness

Conditioning often encourages us to hold in our stomach muscles either for the sake of appearance or to distance our thoughts and feelings from our lower parts. But we should rather be like the animals. Let your spine relax and your belly hang down. Then energy and blood will circulate naturally in your abdomen and you will develop a strong centre. In Japan the belly is known as the "Hara" (see Chapter 3). Holding your belly in is a sign of tension. Whenever you find yourself doing it, breathe out, relax, and let go.

The natural crawl

Crawling is something many of us have not done for years. Even in childhood, many of us were encouraged too quickly through this important stage, which is now thought to influence the development of intelligence. Children are praised for each early step and in this manner proceed through schooling and adult, career-oriented lives favouring the intellect and "higher" things, weakening their relationship with the ground at each stage. We must "stand on our own two feet", become "upright citizens", "walk tall", "make it to the top", and so on. Unfortunately we may have to stiffen up to meet these expectations. So it can be a relief to get down and practise crawling again.

Begin slowly from the previous exercise. You know how to do it! Crawl naturally around the room, noticing how you keep your balance on three limbs as you raise and move the fourth one. If you crawl very slowly, even stop and move backward, you will discover something very important for shiatsu – the ability to increase or reduce your weight through one limb just by moving from your centre.

SITTING AND SQUATTING

For people in much of the world, sitting and squatting on the ground are familiar positions. Work in the fields, cooking, eating, craftwork, and ceremonial activities involve continual squatting, bending, and kneeling. Our more sedentary lifestyle has made these positions alien and difficult. Sitting at desks and working with modern appliances and machines, especially computers, is the cause of many problems of the back, abdomen, and pelvis. Practise kneeling and squatting – they are good for you.

The Seiza posture

Seiza is the natural sitting position for the Japanese in daily life activities, which are traditionally organized at floor level. This sitting position also has formal connotations. Japanese people sit in seiza before performing martial arts, during the tea ceremony, or for Zen meditation where the object is "just to sit". It provides a stable base and is easy to return to, and move from. When sitting still, the feet act like a cushion that lifts the back and helps keep the spine straight. For these reasons many prefer it to the cross-legged position of other traditional cultures. It is the best position for beginning shiatsu because other kneeling or squatting positions flow naturally from it.

Kneeling in seiza

Seiza – alternative position ("sonkyo")

Kneel with your back relaxed but straight, buttocks resting on your heels, feet together (see left), or between your spread heels, toes pointing inward. The variation (see left) with the toes tucked up and under gives you higher support, and makes a change. If your knees are stiff, practise kneeling on a cushion or rolled blanket.

The squatting positions below are simple ways to increase or maintain your flexibility. Any style is beneficial. You can practise them while you chat to friends or watch television.

Half-kneeling position

Toe-raised squat

Flat-foot squat

Low standing exercises

We feel understandably protective of the body's lower regions, but many of us become tense and "closed off" from our lower selves. Sitting with the thighs crossed demonstrates this need for protection. Such habits do nothing for the posture or circulation. The exercises on this page open the groin and encourage blood to flow to the organs and muscles of the lower abdomen and pelvic floor. However, these low stretches are strenuous and demanding. Do them carefully and follow the directions given. Only move on to the more demanding positions shown on page 33 when you are fully comfortable in those shown below.

The low standing stretch

Stand with your feet comfortably wide, toes pointing slightly out. Support the weight of your upper body by leaning forward on to your thighs with your arms fully extended. Sink your bottom lower until your knees make right angles. Relax and breathe into your belly.

Figure-of-eight rotation

Gentle, swaying figure-of-eight rotations with both arms on one knee (here, the left), help to loosen your hips, knees, and ankles as you relax into the position.

Wide stretch 1

From the low standing stretch, turn your right foot out, pivoting on the heel, and the left heel out, pivoting on the ball of your left foot. Now turn to face right, bring your left hand over and lean with both arms on your thigh. Keep your trunk upright, open your chest, and lift your spine; gaze forward and breathe fully. Tighten your back knee gently and look up (see left). Hold for a few seconds, then relax, turn through the centre, and repeat on the other side.

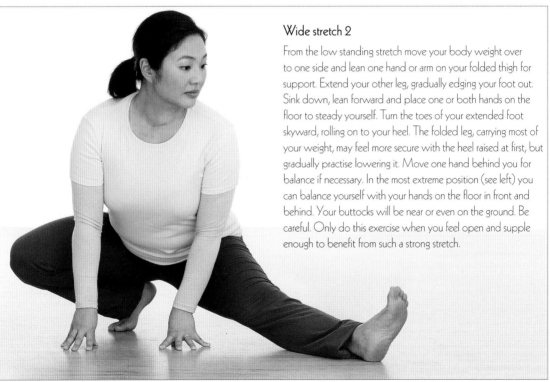

Wide stretch 2

From the low standing stretch move your body weight over to one side and lean one hand or arm on your folded thigh for support. Extend your other leg, gradually edging your foot out. Sink down, lean forward and place one or both hands on the floor to steady yourself. Turn the toes of your extended foot skyward, rolling on to your heel. The folded leg, carrying most of your weight, may feel more secure with the heel raised at first, but gradually practise lowering it. Move one hand behind you for balance if necessary. In the most extreme position (see left) you can balance yourself with your hands on the floor in front and behind. Your buttocks will be near or even on the ground. Be careful. Only do this exercise when you feel open and supple enough to benefit from such a strong stretch.

HAND EXERCISES

Our fingers, hands, and wrists are our main tools in shiatsu. Their strength and flexibility are particularly important. The exercises below, familiar to musicians, sportspeople, and masseurs alike, can be practised in any way: as part of a complete body routine; as a sequence on their own; or singly at any time. Try them while waiting for a bus or train and ignore strange looks from passers-by!

Keep your mind on your posture even while concentrating on your hands. Relax your shoulders and try not to frown, grit your teeth, or hold your breath. Ease up and relax. Give your hands a good shake now and then, between exercises. Remember, they hold tension just as much as any other part of the body does.

Stretching the wrists

Sitting comfortably, bring your palms together close to your chest, fingers pointing upward. Press your hands together and push your wrists down to stretch them (top). Relax, and repeat once or twice. Then turn your hands to point down and stretch by pushing the wrists upward (bottom).

Stretching fingers and palms

Relax your shoulders. Next, interlock your fingers, turn your hands out, and stretch your fingers, palms, and wrists by extending your arms.

Flexing the wrists

Move your wrists from side to side, up and down, then flip them over, palms facing up (supination), and flip them back, palms down (pronation). Then move your hands in any of these ways, in the same or opposite directions, repeating them first slowly, then quickly. Keep your arms relaxed while you do this.

Working on the fingers

Fingers are used in special ways in the practice of shiatsu. They need strength, flexibility, and a relaxed sensitivity. You need to lean your weight through the fingers and thumbs in most shiatsu techniques, rather than simply press with the fingers. Often, too, you use the fingers to provide stability while leaning through the thumbs. More importantly, the fingers are for feeling and will tell you about the physical and "energetic" condition of the people you work with.

1. Loosening the fingers

Extend your fingers one at a time, then grasp each one in turn by the tip, and stretch it back. Hold it for a moment. Then rotate or "stir" each finger in turn around the knuckle joint.

2. Widening the span

To increase the reach of your fingers, insert your fist between each of the fingers of your other hand.

3. Stretching the fingers

Open the space between your thumb and first finger by pressing them together as shown.

Strengthening the fingers

A classic strengthening exercise for thumbs and fingers. Just lean your weight forward for a minute or two, supporting yourself on your outstretched fingers and thumbs.

Gripping and opening

Hold your hands in front of you, and slowly clench your fists as though crushing rocks into powder. Then open them slowly as though against enormous pressure. Repeat a few times. Then open and close your fists lightly and rapidly as a contrast. Ask yourself: did you stop breathing, pull faces, clench your teeth, or tighten your shoulders? Relax, it will come.

BREATHING

Tension, anxiety, and shock restrict the movement of the diaphragm and rib muscles and can inhibit the respiratory mechanism. Consequent shallow breathing limits your energy. The exercises that follow counteract this restriction and will enable you to work more strongly with your breath, increasing the power of your movements. All these exercises begin from a standing position. With your feet firmly planted on the "Earth" you can reach up into "Heaven's Realm", which is traditionally associated with Ki in Oriental medicine. The Lungs circulate this vital energy through the Channels to all parts of the body, through the diaphragm and into the belly, or Hara (see page 51), where it is concentrated at the vital centre known in Japan as the "Tanden". This is the equivalent of the centre of gravity in the physical body. The energies of Heaven and Earth unite here to bring power, harmony, and spontaneity to our actions.

The bow

The bow posture stretches open the chest and diaphragm. Stand firmly, feet apart, knees slightly bent, and support your back by placing your fists or palms wherever feels most comfortable. Bend backward from your hips, making a smooth curve with your back — like a bow. Keep your gaze straight ahead: looking upward distracts and uproots you. Inhale and exhale deeply, opening your chest, diaphragm, and belly. Your lower back and your shoulders will tend to tighten up; try to relax them and keep your shoulders down. After a minute or so, straighten up gently and move slowly into the full forward bend (see opposite). The two exercises are complementary and will increase your energy levels.

The half bend

Stand with feet a shoulder-width apart, knees relaxed. Slowly raise your arms above your head. Look up. Point your fingers inward and keep your elbows curved, so that your arms form a circle around your head. Then breathe out smoothly and, keeping your legs straight but not locked tight, fold at the hips until your trunk is horizontal, with your arms still extended in front (see left). Pause, breathe smoothly, and look out between your hands. Lift and open your chest. After a few breaths, exhale and continue down into a forward bend. Relax.

The forward bend

This is a relaxing position. Make no effort other than to breathe deeply into your Hara. Let your head hang from your neck and your arms hang loosely from your shoulders. Bend your knees slightly. Relax further and sink lower with each exhalation. Keep your weight evenly distributed over your heels and toes. Slowly uncurl when you are ready.

1

2

3

4

5

6

Carrying the circle

With feet apart, gently adopt the forward bend (see position 1, left). With your elbows relaxed and slightly bent, imagine that your arms are encircling a ball of energy, which is recharged every time you breathe in. Keep your feet firmly planted and think of the Earth giving you support, or uplift, as well as a stable base for movement as you lightly carry your "Ki circle" up, around and down.

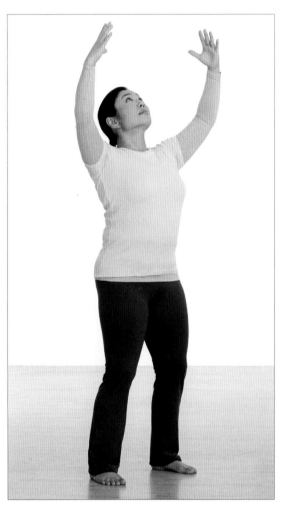

From the forward bend position (1), exhaling gently, turn your trunk to the right, leaning your weight over your right foot (2). Breathe in slowly and deeply and raise your body (3), lifting your circle out and up, until you are upright, gazing skyward between your fingers (see right). Exhale and turn your body slowly to face left (4). Inhale, and on a long exhalation, fold at the hips, weight over your left foot, and carry the circle lightly down, extending your arms and body to the left (5 and 6). Inhale again at the bottom (1). Complete two or three circles in each direction, finishing in the forward bend (1). Release your arms and uncurl into the upright position.

Unifying the mind, body, and breath

As you learn to coordinate your breath and your body movement, you will find that you can work slowly, smoothly, and with the minimum of effort. This is one of the basic principles of the Chinese exercise systems known as Daoyin and Qigong: it is movement from a relaxed state of mind. The mind, remaining calm, centred, and detached, directs the Ki, which influences the physical attributes of the body. The mind harmonizes the breath with the body movement, and this harmony is the path to inner health. The Qigong tradition teaches that "The Mind controls the Ki, Ki moves but the Mind does not move". The simplest method used in Qigong to achieve this stillness of mind is to listen to the sound of your breathing, to concentrate on your body movements as you do them, and to gaze toward the far horizon (whether you are inside or outside), without attaching your mind to external objects.

Stand on the Earth, support the Sky

From the outside this posture is static, but as you concentrate on the supportive Ki of the Earth you will feel the internal dynamic of the exercise. Allow this quality to move right through you, adding power to your arms in supporting the Sky.

Raise your arms slowly on an inhalation and turn your palms skyward so that they are pressing gently upward (see right). Alternatively you can move straight into this exercise from the highest position in "Carrying the circle" (see opposite): just turn your wrists to move your hands into position. Relax your elbows and knees, bending them slightly.

Breathe in Heaven's Ki. As you exhale, direct it to your feet and palms. Support the Sky, without effort. After a while, let go. Lower your arms, and relax (see far right). Stand quietly, breathing calmly for a few minutes.

> "Empty yourself of everything and let the mind be at peace."
> TAO TE CHING,
> LAO TZU

3.PRINCIPLES & TECHNIQUES

Whatever our work, we need the best tools available. The better their quality and accuracy, the more pleasant the task, and the more effective the outcome. Shiatsu is enjoyable, interesting, and rewarding, but it is work nonetheless. Your "tools" are the parts of your body, mainly hands and fingers, and you are the instrument that coordinates them. This chapter will familiarize you with new ways of using your body – rather like a manual for adjusting a fine instrument. The I Ching (Book of Changes) tells us that perseverance brings success; it suggests that we take time and seek help on the way. Use this chapter often as a source of reference as you work through the book.

The special techniques and principles of shiatsu allow us to use the physical body effectively without strain or tiredness. The basic shiatsu techniques for giving pressure (see pp. 42–47) allow us to transmit Ki through the body to our partners. The stretches and rotations that follow (see pp. 48–49) open the Channels and loosen the joints, which improves the flow of Ki. By learning and practising the more advanced techniques explained in the last part of the chapter (see pp. 50–53) you can develop the subtle qualities that bring natural power and vitality to your shiatsu.

At a practical level remember you will need a few "accessories". First, the floor. Work on something firm but comfortable, a thick carpet or folded blanket is fine, but the traditional Japanese three-layer "futon" mattress is ideal for shiatsu. Use a flat pillow for your partner's head, a few cushions for ankles and knees, and a quiet space if you can find one. That's all.

TOOLS AND TECHNIQUES

You can use almost every part of your body in your shiatsu practice. All shiatsu techniques involve gently leaning your body weight through your fingers, thumbs, palms, elbows, knees, or feet. Effective shiatsu depends on the way you apply pressure through these parts on to your partner. The illustrations from this page to page 47 demonstrate shiatsu techniques for applying pressure with each part of your body.

Palming

Palming is one of the simplest and most commonly used shiatsu techniques. It means "leaning" or "holding" with the open palm. Palm pressure is gentle but firm; it is supportive, comforting, and tonifying – encouraging Ki to flow and restoring circulation to areas of underlying weakness. Use the palming technique to soothe away stiffness and defensive reactions in each part of the body before continuing your work with the thumbing technique (see facing page).

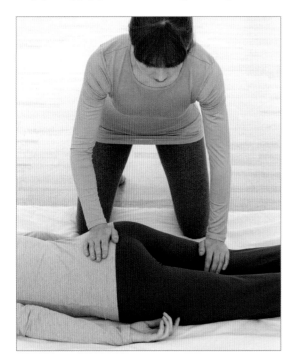

1 Palming the inner leg

Cover the area on your partner's body with your open hand. Bring your body weight slightly forward through your palm. Lean back to slide your hand a little further along, and lean again. Let it follow the shape of your partner's body. With practice you will lean to emphasize your pressure with different parts of your hand. Palming can be given either moving one hand at a time or both together.

2 Palming the back

First principles of pressure

Teachers of the Zen style of shiatsu remind us to use body weight without pressing. "Lean, don't press," they say, yet shiatsu is always described in terms of pressure. It is difficult to think of pressure that is not "pressing". To give good shiatsu you should lean and let your body weight work for you, rather than push or press. Masunaga described this as "penetrating pressure", which combined three elements of technique: perpendicular pressure, stationary pressure, and supporting pressure (see pp. 46–47). It has nothing to do with force or effort; it is something that allows the Ki of the giver and receiver to interact.

Listening to your partner

The best way to "listen" or tune yourself to your partner's Ki while applying pressure is to pay attention to their breathing – sometimes shallow, sometimes deeper, sometimes held, or released with a sigh. Relax and let yourself be taught by what you feel. Then you can move on.

Thumbing

The thumb is more penetrating, precise, and generally more stimulating than the palm. It is the "finger" most commonly used in shiatsu. Always use the thumb extended: think of it as a direct continuation of the line of your arm. Do not bend the thumb at the first joint, or use the muscles of the thumb to press the point (see bottom right). Both detract from sensitivity and feeling, make you tired, and are likely to produce too weak or too strong a pressure, depending on your own strength.

Thumbing

Give pressure by leaning your weight through the thumb tip, a strong technique, or by holding the ball of the thumb rather more flat, which is milder. Steady the thumb by extending the fingers (see above). Never use it on its own. Note: always keep your nails short for your shiatsu sessions.

Using the fingers

Use the fingers for delicate and precise work on the face. Each hand can work on either side of the mid line. Using both hands together gives a feeling of stability.

Thumb and finger

The thumb and finger can be used together when two close points are treated at once, usually along either side of the body's mid line — on the head, the neck, the spine or the sacral region. The thumb and finger are particularly useful when the other hand is being used for support, as shown here.

Thumb and knuckle

This is a more robust alternative to the thumb and finger technique, especially if your fingers are long. It is suited to working down either side of the spine of a muscular back with one hand. Use the knuckle or middle section of the folded forefinger to match the pressure given by the ball of the thumb.

"Dragon's Mouth"

The "Dragon's Mouth" technique is particularly useful for work along the edge of the forearm. The fingers and thumb provide stability on either side of the arm; by a small forward-rolling motion of your wrist you apply precise pressure through the knuckle at the base of the forefinger.

Using the elbows, knees, and feet

There are three reasons for using the elbows, knees, and feet. First, thumbs and fingers can get tired from the physical demands of shiatsu. Second, elbows, knees, and feet are suited to work on stronger or more robust people and parts of the body. The third reason is that elbows and knees are excellent for working into stiff or painful muscles associated with tension. Using the elbows or knees in this way is know as "sedation technique". It enables you to penetrate the areas of blocked Ki in a "friendly" way, dispersing it and reducing pain. The heel of the hand can be used to similar effect.

Elbow technique is very versatile. It can be used on the shoulders, the back, buttocks, hips, thighs, lower legs, and sometimes even the arms.

The only foot techniques described in this book are specifically for working on the receiver's feet. They are safe, easy to practise and very pleasant to receive, and provide the giver with a welcome break from the ground.

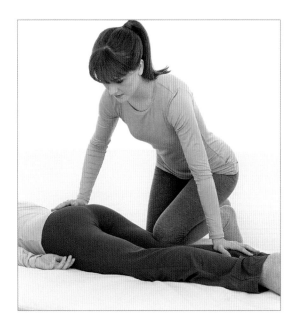

The knees

Knee technique, used mainly on the legs, particularly the thighs, demands good balance and a relaxed body. Support yourself comfortably on all fours, hands in contact with the receiver. Then take more weight on to your hands and raise one knee into position, slowly transferring your weight on to that knee so the receiver experiences comfortable pressure.

The elbows

Before you begin, use your fingers to feel the shape and condition of the area you are working on, then locate your elbow comfortably with their help. Hold your own arms open at the elbow and work with the flattened underside of the angle, not on the "points". Lean without pressing.

Standing on your partner's feet

Either stand with your own heels on your partner's feet (facing away from them), or use the balls of your feet (see above). Keep part of each foot in touch with the ground. Transfer your weight gradually on to their feet. Shift from foot to foot to find comfortable positions.

Body leaning

By leaning your whole body (as shown on this and the facing page), you are using all three elements of penetrating pressure (see below). The exercises shown on these pages are designed to help you understand the difference between leaning and pressing.

PENETRATING PRESSURE

The elements of pressure outlined on page 43 are described in greater detail below.

Perpendicular pressure

Always keep a right angle between the direction of your pressure and your partner's body. This is the Yang component of penetrating pressure; the best way to contact the Ki – straight in.

Stationary pressure

Leaning your body weight without moving is a more passive, receptive, Yin aspect of shiatsu. When your hands are still you can tune into your partner's Ki. You need do nothing – the Ki will respond because its nature is to move. Any extra movements you make may obscure this response.

Leaning on a wall

You can experience secure leaning very easily. Pick a good wall and lean on it to your heart's content — and feel the support.

Shoulder leaning

These simple shoulder-leaning techniques contain the three elements of penetrating pressure: perpendicular, stationary, and support pressure. Ask your partner to sit cross-legged on a cushion, or kneel as shown, firmly planted and secure.

Shoulder leaning (alternative version)

Then relax your weight, leaning at right angles, on to your partner's shoulders. Be aware of the support that they, in turn, are giving you. Support your partner's back with your thigh or knee (see above). You should both be comfortable. Try leaning on your elbows on different parts of the shoulders (see above left).

Supporting pressure

You are already familiar with the idea of the ground as your support (see pp. 26–29). Supporting pressure is both a technique in which we support our partner, and a quality of touch that conveys care, consideration, and safety. It is another hidden, Yin, Earth-related aspect of good shiatsu.

The support hand

This provides a balance for the pressure being applied with the working hand (see "The use of two hands connecting", p. 50). Sometimes we use the whole body to provide support, particularly for shiatsu in the sitting position.

Mutual support

You will be supported not only by the ground but by the receiver's body. The degree to which you trust in your receiver's physical strength and support will determine the quality of energy they get from you. Support is a two-way process. This leads to a mutual trust that allows relaxation – and this is the moment that leads to change, brought about by the free movement of Ki in your partner's body. The Japanese character for "human being" is like two sticks supporting each other. It conveys the fundamental point that human beings need each other.

Crawling on to your partner's back

Make your partner comfortable on a blanket or carpeted floor. Start from the basic crawling position and move your hands on to the strong parts of your partner's back — the thoracic vertebrae and the sacral region (see above), or the buttocks.
Bring your weight forward slowly until your arms are at right angles to your partner. Lean, applying perpendicular, supporting pressure. Pause for a moment, allowing the stationary aspect of your pressure to penetrate. Let your own spine relax, and take a breath. Then ease back, move your hands into another comfortable position and lean once more. Your partner will often exhale deeply with your pressure. Don't be afraid — they will breathe in again when they want to.

Leaning on your partner

This exercise in mutual support subtly blends all three aspects of penetrating pressure. Sitting back to back, cross-legged or with your legs outstretched, bend forward a little and edge close together. Uncurl and adjust your backs to fit each other as well as possible. If you agree that neither of you feel burdened but both feel supported, just relax, be aware of each other's breathing, lean on each other, and "merge" awhile.

STRETCHES AND ROTATIONS

These are an important part of your shiatsu technique. Rotations loosen the joints and position the limbs correctly for working on each Channel. Stretches open up the Channel, activating the Ki; this makes diagnosis easier and treatment more effective.

Stiff and painful joints are the result of blockages in the circulation of Ki and Blood, which do not flow with great ease at the joints, owing to the density of ligaments and tendons that surround the bones. For this reason rotations and stretches are a particularly valuable aspect of treatment.

Once you have practised the exercises shown here for a while, try to incorporate the principles of advanced shiatsu technique (see pp. 50–53), especially "Keeping your Hara open" and "Visualizing circles".

Arm rotation

Widen your stance for this technique, keeping your nearside knee on the ground and raising the other knee to place your foot on the floor. Grasp firmly round the top of your partner's shoulder with your near-side hand and pick up the wrist with your other, gently shaking the arm to loosen the elbow.

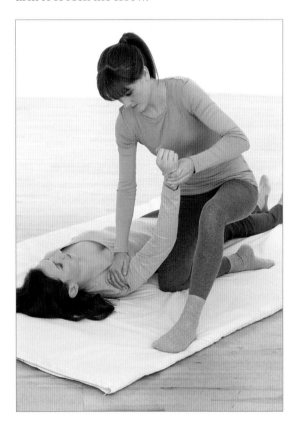

Rotating the arm

Make a number of circling movements, by carrying the wrist forward, over and above the shoulder, then out to the side and back toward you, gently pulling on your partner's wrist and shoulder to stretch all the joints.
Practise widening the circle toward a full stretch. Move your whole body to follow the action.

Leg rotations

Rotating the leg at the hip, knee, or ankle joints involves many variations of technique depending on which joint is being worked and on the position of the receiver. They are described in detail in the practical routines later in the book. The leg is heavy, so you must always make certain to have a wide base.

Rotating the leg

Relax your limbs and lift from underneath (see "Relax and keep weight underside" p. 52). Don't strain or pull up from your back.

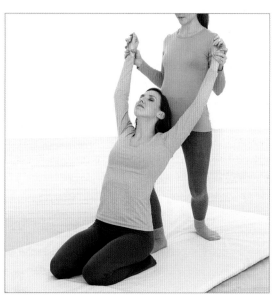

Full body stretch

Side position stretch

Stretches

These are often incorporated into the rotations, merely by pausing and stretching the limb at a number of points in the circle. Done carefully and without force, they release tension and blockages. They also inform you more fully about the receiver's condition. Lax movements indicate lack of muscle tone or deficient Ki. Tightness or stiffness indicates a local blockage of Ki. Full body stretches (see above) are often used once or twice in a session to release Ki generally and help the receiver to relax.

PRINCIPLES OF ADVANCED TECHNIQUE

From the basic principles and techniques, you can move on to deepen your understanding of the subtle qualities of good shiatsu. This will enhance the experience for the receiver as well as your ability as a practitioner. Absorbing these subtle techniques produces great Ki power but can take years of practice. However, one must start sometime and you are in good company – in Zen there are no experts, only beginners.

The use of two hands connecting

This principle, developed by Masunaga, is a unique distinguishing feature of Zen shiatsu. Shiatsu encompasses support, a Yin quality; and movement, a Yang, dynamic aspect. Our two hands harmonize the Yin, supportive, and Yang, dynamic, aspects of our work. With practice we begin to feel their unifying power in our partner's response. One hand fulfils the supporting function for both giver and receiver (see "The support hand" on p. 47). Remaining stationary, it contacts the receiver's "centres of energy" and is sometimes called the "listening" or "parent" hand. The other, more active hand, sometimes known as the "child", follows the

> *Shiatsu masters say: "Two hands feel like one" – the receiver feels something whole and complete. This is good shiatsu.*

Ki in its movement round the body, innocently exploring the receiver's condition. Either hand can play the supporting roles as required, the important thing being that parent and child are "in touch" with each other (see below).

Continuity

A feeling of flow and continuity is essential to enhance your partner's experience of shiatsu. Continuity depends on your movements and the focus of your mind.

Concentrate on the fluent use of your hands as you work around your partner's body. Follow the Ki in its Channels by sliding your active hand along without breaking contact, to feel its condition and locate the tsubos. Move or pause as necessary and always maintain

Two hands connecting

contact with your support hand. Focus your attention on your partner's breathing, and work from your Hara (see below).

When your body and mind act in concert, your partner will be unaware of your technique but will experience the shiatsu as being deeply appropriate. Good continuity depends on your ability to work from the Hara.

Hara awareness

The Hara is the belly or abdomen. It is regarded not only as the physical centre of gravity but as the the seat of your constitutional energy or life force, both the origin of Ki and the place where it returns. In Japan, to "have a good Hara" means to be in good health, to have vitality. To be "in Hara" means to be aware of yourself, coordinated and relaxed.

When our breathing is deep and easy, the lower Hara is naturally nourished by the breath and revitalized and supported by good digestion and proper rest. Tension in the chest and diaphragm prevent this smooth downward connection. To practise leading

your own breath smoothly down, concentrate first on breathing out fully. Pause and relax at the end of the exhalation, and observe how your diaphragm works spontaneously as the in-breath comes by itself (see also the exercise on p. 87).

Working from the Hara

In practice the Hara is the centre of action. To "move from your Hara" is the epitome of good shiatsu. You can learn to move from your Hara by following "Keeping your Hara open" and "Keeping your weight underside" on page 52. The exercises in Chapter 2 for grounding and breathing will help you to develop Hara consciousness.

The Hara region becomes the focus of touch diagnosis as we develop – but for now, sitting in Hara, and just touching your partner's Hara is enough; a powerfully simple technique.

The Tanden and the Mei Mon

The centre of the Hara is a point the width of three fingers below the navel. It is known as the Tanden, or "Sea of Ki". A corresponding point, connected to the Tanden via the Kidneys is the Mei Mon, located in the centre of the spine, between the second and the third lumbar vertebrae. Also known as "Life Gate" or the "Gate of the Fire of Vitality", the Mei Mon is the seat of Kidney Yang (see p. 77).

Sitting in Hara

Relax and keep the weight underside

The most important principle of shiatsu is to relax. This does not mean flopping or collapsing, it is merely a reminder to work without effort. Never hunch your back or raise your shoulders and always relax your elbows. Take the easy way and allow your Ki to work for you; it will, if you stay in your Hara.

Relaxation connects you with the ground. Keeping weight underside, a principle borrowed from Aikido, is a way of conveying the energy of the ground through your body.

Keeping the weight underside

Whatever your position, imagine the upper side of your body or limbs are light and the lower aspects heavy – as though being pulled toward Earth. For example: when extending your arm to work with fingers, thumb, or palm, be aware of the heaviness of your elbow. Being "grounded" in this way allows you to draw energy from the Earth up through your body along all the heavier parts. Lightly direct your Ki with your mind and let the Earth provide both uplift and pulling power. This is the essence of relaxed shiatsu.

Keeping your Hara open

Your aim as a practitioner is to keep your Hara open in all your movements. You can learn to do this by keeping a wide base when giving shiatsu; even in seiza position (see p. 30), have at least the width of a fist between your knees. In this way your actions will flow more easily from the Tanden and you will keep in touch with the receiver's Ki. By keeping your centre of gravity in your Hara, you will also be able to work without losing your balance. The position of your arms is just as important. If you work

Keeping the Hara open and visualizing circles

too closely you will weaken your Ki power and compensate by using muscular strength, which will tire you.

Visualizing circles

Ki is best conveyed along smooth, open curves. Imagine a flexible sphere in front of your body, encompassed by your arms and chest, and smaller circles supporting your armpits, keeping all the joints open and soft. These will help foster your Ki and at the same time keep your Hara open.

Finding the correct position

By combining all the principles outlined in this chapter your shiatsu will become an efficient, effective, and enjoyable occupation. All the principles apply at every moment. Practise incorporating them as you work on your partner's body. Then you will naturally begin to find the right position for you. If you forget the principles you are more likely to make hard work of your shiatsu. There is no absolutely correct posture but the principles are a guide by which you can monitor yourself. The illustrations on this page highlight the difference between working with these principles and trying to work without them.

The Hara at the centre of gravity

In the illustration (see above, top), the giver is over-extending his body, which leads to strain. His work may feel inconsistent and unsettling. By stepping out to create a wide base (see above), the Hara is at his centre of gravity, as it should be. He can lean with perpendicular pressure from a comfortable position.

Working from a wide base

Without a wide base (see above, top), and too close to his partner, the giver hunches his back, leading to backache. He cannot thumb correctly because his arm and thumb are bent. He "presses" with his thumb. In the correct position (see above) the giver is balanced and comfortable and works with his thumb and fingers extended. His work will feel more "connected".

4.THE BASIC SHIATSU ROUTINE

The active partner is the "giver" of shiatsu from a practical point of view, but communication through physical contact goes both ways. Your hands work and "listen". You gain a degree of physical support from your partner and respond intuitively to his or her feelings, which means that you both give and receive at the same time.

Similarly, when you receive shiatsu, you also participate in a two-way process. Allow yourself to feel and respond naturally to any sensations or emotions that arise, and consciously "let go" into the experience. You may feel tense. Sometimes shiatsu can border on the painful, but is should feel like good or helpful pain, never more. Breathe naturally when you feel the pressure and let the tension flow away. Your partner will learn to follow your breathing. Traditionally, learning to receive shiatsu is said to take almost as long as learning to give it.

The best shiatsu sessions are often relaxed, quiet, with few words, but feel free to talk if it seems appropriate. Both the giver and the receiver should give feedback if there is any discomfort or tension. Either partner may have spontaneous insights during a session – share them, they may be valuable; but don't let talking interrupt the continuity.

The basic routine is summarized on pages 56–63. Read the whole chapter before you attempt it. Then, introduce your partner to the space you have prepared for the session and explain what you are going to do. Even if they are already familiar with shiatsu, this ritual will put you both at ease. Ask briefly how your partner is feeling. If you are a bit nervous yourself, why not admit it? A frank exchange of your feelings can ease the situation. Later, your nervousness will disappear. Invite your partner to lie down, then you can begin.

BEGINNING THE BASIC ROUTINE

In the first part of your shiatsu session you will be working with your partner lying face down – the "prone" position. Starting with the back, then the buttocks, the legs, and the feet, you return to the shoulders to finish. Make your partner comfortable, their arms down at their sides so the shoulders rest easily on the floor. A few people will need a pillow in this position (see p. 63) but most will be comfortable with the head turned to one side: remind them to turn it to the other side from time to time to prevent the neck from becoming stiff. Invite them to let you know if you lean or press too hard, as well as to tell you if any place feels particularly good. You can learn a lot from a little feedback.

Working on the back

Most people experience the back and shoulders as a safe part of the body to receive contact. The area is structurally strong, and the Yang Channels, associated with the body's defence, flow downward through it.

Many people suffer from backache, or tension in the shoulders, due to overwork and tiredness. Your partner's back can take your weight and, by leaning on it, you will help them "let go" and release tension from tired, aching muscles.

Preparation: Stimulating the Ki

Sit in seiza posture next to your partner, if necessary moving their arm a little away from their side to make room for yourself. Breathe into your Hara. Hold your hands at chest level and rub them together briskly and firmly for 30–40 seconds, keeping your shoulders relaxed.

This will stimulate the flow of Ki in your whole body, and will warm and sensitize your hands at the start of a session.vKeep your hands joined and your attention focused on how you are feeling for a moment, before making contact with your partner.

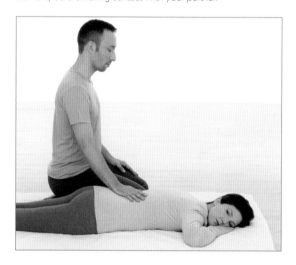

1. Making the first contact

When you are ready, simply rest your hand on any part of your partner's lumbar (lower back) region. Spend a few moments holding your palm gently in place, giving your partner time to adjust to your contact. Start to focus your attention on the depth and rhythm of your partner's breathing.

Contact the upper and lower spine

Kneel up, and, with your hand still in contact, turn to face your partner's body. Reposition your hands, one in the sacral region and the other on the back of the chest (thoracic region, see p. 47). Lean forward. Let your spine relax, breathe easily and continue to focus on your partner's breathing for a few moments.

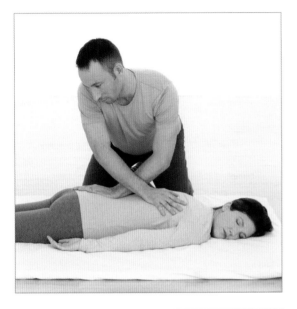

2. Lumbar cross stretch

Use the following technique to open the lumbar curve and ease tight muscles before putting direct pressure on the back. Shift your weight back into your hips and knees and bring your upper hand down to the buttock/hip region on the side nearest you. Move your lower hand up to the rib margin on the far side. Lean forward again and use your body weight to create a stretch between your crossed hands. It may help to ask your partner to exhale as you do this.

Hold for a moment, then ease back slightly and bring your hands, one at a time, across to the opposite corresponding positions and repeat the stretch. Do this twice on both sides.

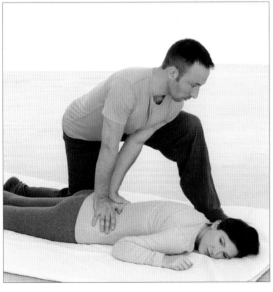

3. The lunge position

Turn to face your partner's head, then place your hands on the upper back, between the shoulder blades, your fingers pointing outward away from each other and the heels of your hands about 1 in (2.5 cm) away from each side of the spine (see p. 42). Move your Hara forward, and lean on to your partner's back, using perpendicular pressure. Now ease back and move your hands down, one at a time. Each time they are level, lean forward again to apply perpendicular pressure.

As you approach the lower spine, move your foot out (see left) to work from a wider base. Sink your weight back, with your arms perpendicular to the lower back and sacro-lumbar region. Lean into the position. Now bring your foot closer to finish with perpendicular pressure on the sacrum. Try to keep these leg movements smooth: your partner will give you the stability you need.

The pelvis and sacro-lumbar region

The area of the buttocks, hips, and pelvis is often affected by stress, poor posture, and a sedentary lifestyle, yet many of us do not recognize the degree to which we accumulate tension here. Tension can produce a misalignment of hips and spine and vice versa.

Basic emotions, such as anger and hatred, affect this area and find expression in kicking and stamping. Our natural sexuality is expressed in pelvic mobility and a natural swinging of the hips. But we restrain all these for much of the time. There are often insufficient healthy avenues for the expression of such natural feelings, but engaging in sports, music, and dancing activities with your friends will help. Shiatsu can relieve many problems that stem from poor circulation in this area, including backache, sciatica, varicose veins, menstrual pain, bladder troubles, and sexual problems in both men and women.

4. Elbowing the buttocks

The buttock (gluteal) muscles are the largest in the body. They hold a lot of tension, and working them with the thumb is tiring — use elbow technique here. Turn to face your partner and support yourself with one hand on the small of the back. With the flattened elbow of your other arm, lean into the buttock on the near side where you can let your weight sink comfortably, and which allows your partner to relax. Then shift your weight forward into the other buttock, feeling your way into those spots that easily take your weight.

5. The sacral squeeze

Still leaning gently on your partner for support, step over their thighs. Interlace your fingers and lean into each side of the sacrum, squeezing with the heels of both hands. Reinforce the action by bringing your body forward; you may find it more comfortable to support one elbow with your leg.

The legs

Improving the energy flow to the legs is an important part of being "grounded". Many people live almost exclusively "in their heads" – unaware of the tension in their leg muscles, which effectively cuts them off from the ground. High-flying achievers often deny themselves the relaxation they need. Dreamers ignore the physical, earth-bound aspects of their reality, and as a result obtain no energy from it, and fail to realize their dreams. Both types may continue in their ways until physical illness demands their attention. Shiatsu can forestall many problems by bringing people back to earth, in touch with their physical body.

Starting the routine

To manage the shiatsu routine on the leg, keep a wide base. Check that your partner's leg is relaxed, the knees and toes turned slightly inward. Place a cushion under the ankles if their legs are stiff.

This is your first chance to practise the principle of "two hands connecting" (see p. 50). Balance and support yourself lightly with one hand on your partner's sacrum and lean forward from your Hara to apply stationary, perpendicular pressure down the leg with the other.

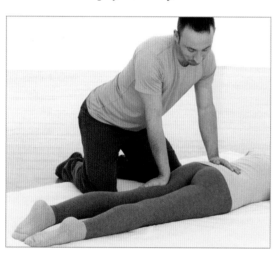

6. Palming the near leg

Lean on to the uppermost part of the thigh. Point the fingers outward to avoid the risk of confusing or upsetting your partner by inadvertently touching their genitals. Work down the middle of the leg, directing your pressure straight into the centre. Move your hand down a few inches at a time, easing back toward your haunches whenever you change position.

7. Working down the lower leg

As you move down the thigh, turn your hand to point the fingers inward. Work gently over the knee. Keeping a wide base, palm down the lower leg to finish above the heel. Apply a medium pressure through the palm or heel of the hand. Keep your hand relaxed to hug the shape of the leg as you proceed (see p. 42). With your support hand still in place, move over to the far side to palm the other leg in the same way. Swap your support hand as you take up your position on the other side.

The three-way stretch

This stretch works on the hip, knee, and ankle joints to release tension and help the flow of Ki down the leg.

8. The three-way stretch

Move back to the first side. With your support hand still resting on the sacrum, reach under your partner's ankle and lift the lower leg, stretching the knee and thigh.

9. The three-way stretch

Fold the foot over toward the centre of the buttock. Lean gently but firmly, then slide your hand toward the toes to stretch the foot. Pause for a moment, then carry the foot back out to release the knee joint (see step 8).

10. The three-way stretch

Fold the leg across to the opposite buttock and stretch, following the movement with your body.

11. The three-way stretch

Release the leg again as in step 8 and carry it round in a circular movement, bringing the foot toward you and along the nearside of your partner's buttock. Then place the foot on the floor, toes pointing slightly inward. Move to the other side and repeat the three-way stretch on the other leg.

The feet

After performing the three-way stretch, it is important to complete the grounding process by working on your partner's feet. The work you have been doing in the routine so far mainly contacts the Yang Ki, which flows in Channels down the back and outside surfaces from the head. Many shiatsu techniques for the feet help balance Yang with Yin in the whole body.

An easy and most effective technique is to walk or stand on your partner's feet. Try walking forward gradually, up on to the soles, leaning slowly first into one foot then the other (see p. 45). Alternatively, back up on to them with your heels. This will give you a rest from kneeling before you begin the next section.

Natural break

Finishing the routine on the feet provides a natural break for both you and your partner. Both of you will enjoy the pause and you can stretch as you move to the top of your partner's body for the next part of the routine. Before starting work on the back and shoulders, suggest that your partner turn to face the other side. A gentle reminder to do this is worthwhile, because a shiatsu session can be so relaxing that people "forget themselves". It is a shame if a stiff neck detracts from the benefits at the end of your session.

Upper back and shoulders

We have all experienced tension in the upper back and shoulders. This last part of the prone routine helps to disperse tension and can also benefit the lungs, easing coughs and tightness in the chest. Use the same natural application of your body weight through simple palm and thumb techniques. Relax into them, enjoy yourself, and allow the pressure to work for both of you.

12. Making contact with the back

Kneel at your partner's head, with your knees apart (a good guide is to place your knees level with your partner's ears), at a comfortable distance from them. Too close and your partner will feel oppressed; too far and you will strain, or your pressure will not be perpendicular. Imagine a working circle (see p. 52); lean comfortably with both hands on the slope of the shoulders. Pause and relax.

13. Palming between the shoulder blades

This technique for palming down the back is similar to the one you have already used (see p. 42). Lean into the muscles about 1 in (2.5 cm) each side of the spine. Begin near the base of the neck, and palm down between the shoulder blades. Move down the back, one hand at a time, and maintain the perpendicular pressure. Work down to the bottom of the shoulder blades. Pressing here will affect your partner's breathing, but keep your movements smooth and your pressure even.

14. Thumbing each side of the spine

Returning to the top of the back, work with both your thumbs down the muscular ridge about 1 in (2.5 cm) each side of the spine. Begin near the most prominent vertebra at the base of the neck and finish level with the base of the shoulder blades.

15. Thumbing across the shoulders

Take a line from the base of the neck along the top of your partner's shoulder. Use the flattened ball of one thumb and work outward in stages to the bony angle at the extremity of the shoulder (see above). Some points may be tender so work carefully. Keep your elbow relaxed and lean in from the hip. Use your other hand for support.

Now take another line about 1 in (2.5 cm) lower, giving thumb pressure outward along the muscle between the top of the shoulder and the bony ridge of the shoulder blade. Repeat a few times on each shoulder.

Note:

The pressure on the chest and ribs in the prone position may be uncomfortable for some people. Others may have difficulty keeping their neck turned fully to the side. In these cases a pillow under the chest (see above) can provide the solution.

Turning over

To finish your prone routine, rest your hands on your partner's upper back for a moment or two and check how she or he is feeling. Then invite your partner to turn over into the supine position. Stay kneeling where you are during this time. Rest your palms on your partner's forehead or temples for a short while, as a gesture of support and to maintain contact during this transitional phase.

THE SUPINE POSITION

Giving shiatsu on the front of the body needs extra consideration. The chest, diaphragm, and belly are centres of emotion and by lying on our backs we are immediately more open, so we may feel exposed and vulnerable. Working face to face can feel intense and involving. Treat your partner with consideration and respect, but continue your shiatsu in an easy, relaxed manner. Good, solid contact can be very strengthening and affirming for your partner. There is no need to be over-cautious.

Hara contact

In this part of the routine, begin by contacting your partner's Hara. Then work on the inner aspect of each arm and hand. Afterwards return to the Hara before giving shiatsu to the legs.

Checking for relaxation

If you feel your partner trying to help you by moving or holding their arm, gently encourage them to "let go" – something you may often have to repeat when you learn to do the full stretches and rotations. Many people find that giving up control to relax with another person is not easy.

1. Hara contact

Sit in seiza at your partner's side. Rest your hand on their Hara with fingertips above, and the heel of the hand below the navel. Relax your arm, do not lean or press. Observe, feel the breathing and just "be" with them for a moment before starting. Even as a beginner, you can contact your partner's Ki at a deep level. The art of simply touching, called Waki, is the essence of shiatsu. We accept the person as they are.

2. Loosening the arm

Pick up your partner's arm by the hand or wrist, move your other hand from their Hara to their shoulder and, by leaning back slightly, stretch the arm out. Now move your near hand from the shoulder to the elbow and, carrying the arm, bend and rotate the forearm.

Yin Channels

The Ki of the Yin Organs circulates on the front of the body and on the inner surfaces of the limbs – the softer parts that we are naturally inclined to protect. The Yin Organs are traditionally associated with the emotions in Oriental medicine.

3. Palming the arm

Place your partner's arm at a right angle to their side. The palm and inner surface of their arm should be facing upward. Then squatting, or kneeling up on your toes, and keeping a wide base, lean with your support hand on to the front of their shoulder. Palm their arm with the other, moving down little by little. Keep both hands relaxed, hugging the shape of the limb.

4. Working on the palm

The Ki is particularly responsive at the hands and feet. Work on the hand is very satisfying and relaxing for the receiver. Give thumb shiatsu to your partner's palm by adopting a special stretching and opening grip: with your partner's fingers toward you, tuck your little fingers through the first space between the

fingers, and finger and thumb, on each side of the hand, supporting the back of your partner's hand with your fingers (see above left). Then work with extended thumbs giving pressure systematically over the whole palm (see above). You can rest the backs of your hands on your knees while you work.

5. Finger pulling

All the main Channels end or begin on the fingers or toes. The shiatsu technique used to stimulate the Channel endings is to squeeze the sides of the finger firmly between your thumb and the knuckle of your index finger. Work along each finger and thumb in stages from knuckle to fingertip.

The Ki finds its own direction

Some styles of shiatsu make a rule of following the direction of the Yin and Yang Channels up and down the limbs to "tonify" the Ki. In the Zen style it is considered more important to keep contact with the centre and work outward. The Yin Channels flow up the inner surface of the legs. Yet we always work down the legs, even though this goes "against the flow" of the Ki in the Yin Channel.

The two hands connect and open the Channels and the Ki moves spontaneously if we make good contact and develop "penetrating pressure". We don't need to tell the Ki where to go. It will go there itself!

6. Palming the near leg

After working on the arms and hands, return to your partner's Hara. Kneel facing inward as close to your partner's body as possible, knees apart. A wide base will help you to work all the way down the leg without over-reaching. Rest one hand comfortably on your partner's Hara and lean the other hand on to the top of the thigh, fingers pointing outward. Kneel up if you need extra height.

Palm the near side of the leg past the knee to the ankle, moving in stages, sliding the hand along between points to keep contact. On the lower leg, give more pressure to the outside of the shinbone through the heel of the hand, fingertips curled naturally over for support (see above).

7. Palming the far leg

Bring your weight forward to palm down the inner aspect of the far leg. Keep the pressure of your support hand constant on the Hara as you rock back and forward to move and give pressure with your active hand. Palm down from thigh to ankle. Then move round to repeat the work on the two aspects of the legs from the other side.

The feet

After palming the legs, move down to the feet. You can finish by simply grasping both feet below the ankle and squeezing all the way down the sides, leaning back and stretching them down a little as you do so. Or you can attempt, with care, and your mind on your Hara, the following stretching and loosening sequence for the waist and lower spine.

8. Raising the feet

Squat down close to your partner's feet, your knees wide outside your arms and your back as straight as possible. Reach down behind your partner's ankles to lift their heels a fraction off the floor. Pause and breathe.

9. Resting on your thighs

In one smooth movement, keeping your back as straight as possible, exhale as you straighten your knees to lift your partner's legs about 30 degrees and step in a little to rest your arms on your thighs (see above). Anchored by your partner's body weight, lean back to stretch the spine, while you relax and breathe. Only when you are comfortable and ready, try the next step: swinging your partner's legs in a wide arc.

10. Swinging the legs

This move loosens the waist and lumbar region — a relief for tired, aching backs. Begin with small side-to-side rocking movements while still supporting your elbows. Then transfer your weight from foot to foot as you swing their legs and push their feet out, up, and away from you on each side — only a few times before resting. Then lower the legs carefully back to the floor. Keep your Hara low and your back straight.

Finishing the routine

The way you finish your shiatsu treatments is as important as the way you begin. There is no set pattern for shiatsu routines. Often we finish on the feet, as in this routine, which is very good for grounding people. But sometimes the hands or the head and neck are the last areas we work. Then, as well as speaking to your partner, use touch to signal the end. A short pause followed by a hand on their shoulder or a squeeze of their wrist conveys the message. Best of all is to contact the Hara. Tell your partner gently that the work is done for now. You may find that they have become very relaxed. Suggest that they open their eyes and re-orient themselves before slowly getting up. Ask them how they feel. Give them time!

5.PATTERNS OF KI

From ancient times the Chinese interpreted the behaviour of Ki from its manifestations. Areas of pain, swelling, irritation, or redness that arose in illness were seen as disturbances or blockages of Ki on the body surface. It was found that some conditions, even internal ones, could be ameliorated by pressing or rubbing these tender areas. Other "points of pain" were discovered in the process that also seemed to bring benefit when pressed.

The use of points was fairly random at first, but certain of them were repeatedly found helpful for similar conditions and, as more were added, they were recorded and systemized. Through experience it became clear that all aspects of the body were interrelated, and the theory arose that the points were linked by a network of subtle interconnecting Channels. These conducted Ki to all parts inside the body and to the skin on the outside. Twelve primary Channels came to be associated with the body's main Organs.

Signs and symptoms of disease can be seen as part of a "pattern of disharmony", manifesting a disturbance of Ki in certain channels and, possibly, a deeper dysfunction in the corresponding organ system. In the holistic (yin-yang) way of thinking of the East, it is impossible to view illness and health separately. Our vital forces, flowing currents of Ki, are constantly adapting to change, but our Ki also follows recurring patterns, which accord with life's rhythms and the body's self-regulating functions. The major phases in this pattern are formally represented by the twelve primary Channels but, in reality, these primary expressions of Ki are subtle, whole body movements arising spontaneously in response to the deepest inner needs of our organism. Reflecting "Kyo-jitsu", the life principle incorporated by Masunaga into his meridian shiatsu method, they can be recognized, and experienced, as corresponding to the archetypal images associated with the twelve channels in their Yin-Yang pairs (opposite).

The major Channels flow near to the surface and can be influenced through shiatsu at points along their path, reharmonizing the Organs and restoring and maintaining balance in the whole system. The study of the Channels, or meridians, is an essential step in transforming your shiatsu from a general treatment, which may be relaxing or stimulating, into a more precise and effective means of healing.

The major Channels are illustrated on pages 70–71, and the nature of the points, or tsubos, is described on page 73. The sequence of the Channels, and the cyclical movement of their Ki are explained on page 74. Pages 76–77 summarize the functions of the Organs.

Lungs and Large Intestine: Breathing, energy exchange; elimination.

Stomach and Spleen: Reaching out for nourishment and nurture; enfolding.

Heart and Small Intestine: Contemplation and assimilation.

Bladder and Kidney: Action — the drive to live, survive and go on.

Pericardium and Triple Burner: Protection at the core and at the surface.

Gall Bladder and Liver: Free-flow — storing and distributing Ki; planning and decisions.

THE MAJOR CHANNELS (THE MERIDIAN NETWORK)

Ki is distributed throughout the body by an intricate web of subtle Channels. Twelve "primary Channels" connect internally with the Organs and circulate the Ki near the surface via pathways that flow in a particular pattern over the head and trunk and along the limbs. Most of the classical pressure points are found along the primary Channels. These Channels are

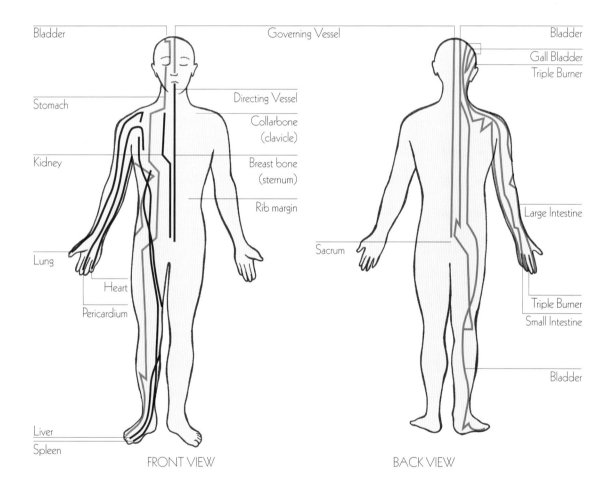

FRONT VIEW

Bladder
Stomach
Kidney
Lung
Heart
Pericardium
Liver
Spleen

Governing Vessel
Directing Vessel
Collarbone (clavicle)
Breast bone (sternum)
Rib margin

BACK VIEW

Bladder
Gall Bladder
Triple Burner
Sacrum
Large Intestine
Triple Burner
Small Intestine
Bladder

70

frequently called "meridians" in the West, and this term may be freely substituted.

The Internal Channels

Each of the twelve main Channels has its interior pathway, connecting the exterior part with its own inner organ as well as its yin or yang paired organ. The inner pathways are also the expression of other vital energetic links within the body, reflecting the strong relationship between the major organs and the sensory organs and representing many subtle connections long understood in Eastern medicine. Thus, for example, the internal pathway of the Liver Channel most clearly shows how the Liver influences such diverse body parts as the genitals and reproductive system, the throat, the eyes and the top of the head, and explains certain symptoms that can appear when the Channel is in disharmony. The Internal Meridian pathways are not much emphasized in shiatsu schools, though they complete the entire system and aid our understanding of how Ki moves in the body – the yin-yang dynamic between the inside and the outside and the upper and lower regions and so on. In this book they are included with the main Channel illustrations in the following chapters, shown as a broken line. Study them at your leisure.

The Central Channels

According to tradition, there are eight "extra Channels", circulating deeper in the body, that intersect with the twelve primary Channels, and act as reservoirs of Ki. Two of these extra Channels, the "mid line" Channels, are of particular importance. They have their own points and are sometimes included with the primary Channels. Together, these fourteen "major Channels" are the subjects of this book.

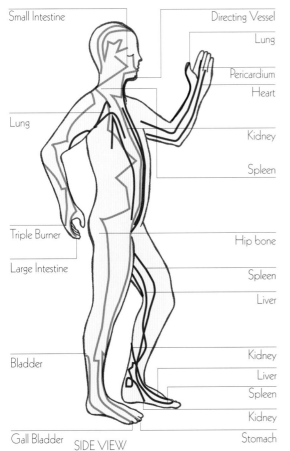

Small Intestine

Lung

Triple Burner

Large Intestine

Bladder

Gall Bladder   SIDE VIEW

Directing Vessel

Lung

Pericardium

Heart

Kidney

Spleen

Hip bone

Spleen

Liver

Kidney

Liver

Spleen

Kidney

Stomach

The superficial pathways of all the major Channels are shown most clearly in the front, back, and side views. The Yin Channels, shown in blue, flow from the feet up to the chest and from the chest out to the fingertips. The Yang Channels, shown in orange, are, with the exception of the Stomach Channel (see p. 84), all located on the back and outer surfaces of the limbs. They flow from the hands to the head and downward to the feet.

The mid line Channels, also known as the "Governing Vessel" and the "Directing Vessel", control all the others. The Governing Vessel runs up the spine and over the head. It controls all the Yang Channels. The Yin Channels are regulated by the Directing Vessel, which follows the mid line over the abdomen and chest up to the throat and mouth. Thumb and finger pressure can be given to points along the mid line Channels, but it is usual to keep in touch with these Channels during a shiatsu session with the support hand (see p. 47). Maintain contact in this way on the Hara, chest, or lower back, while the active hand works outward from these areas. By keeping the support hand on the mid-line, we can "tune in" to the central circulation of Ki while we work on the primary Channels.

Key to Channel abbreviations used in the book

Bl	Bladder
DV	Directing Vessel
GB	Gall Bladder
GV	Governing Vessel
H	Heart
K	Kidney
LI	Large Intestine
Liv	Liver
Lu	Lung
P	Pericardium
SI	Small Intestine
Sp	Spleen
St	Stomach
TB	Triple Burner

Naming the Channels

The full name for each Channel is derived from the Organ to which it is connected, the limb along which it runs, the time of its activity according to the Chinese Clock (see p. 75), its position on the arm or leg, and its polarity (Yin or Yang). So, for example, the full name for the Lung Channel is Lung Channel, arm Greater Yin.

Classical points

Nearly all of the 365 classical points or tsubos, situated along the 14 Channels, were established by the time of *The Yellow Emperor's Classic of Internal Medicine* – the earliest Chinese medical work. Over centuries of experience these became recognized for their predictable influence over certain functions and parts of the body.

Some points reacted to certain diseases, becoming irritated, and tender when pressed. Because of this, they could be used for diagnosis as well as treatment. Groups of points with similar characteristics were subsequently linked, and the system of Channels became established.

However, the older system of treating any points of pain or tenderness remained in the tradition. The Chinese call these points "Ah Shi" points, meaning "that's it!", as a response to touching the affected part. Shiatsu treatment is not confined to classical acupuncture points: look for the "hollows" or points of deepest penetration that feel satisfying to the receiver. This is where you can work on the Ki.

Tsubos

A tsubo is a pressure point, where the Ki can gather – a "hollow" or "opening" where the Ki can be reached and influenced by applying pressure. Its structure is more three-dimensional than the word "point" suggests. Both Channels and tsubos are found in the spaces between the muscles and other tissues of the body.

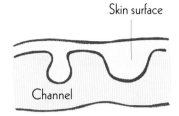

Skin surface

Channel

Normal tsubos

Tsubos are like openings into the Channel. Your pressure is accepted. Ki responds. Your partner feels comforted and supported. Even pain is pleasant pain. Some tsubos are more lax, or open, than others.

Blocked tsubos

Physical tension blocks Ki and produces distorted or closed tsubos that are difficult to penetrate (see pp. 158–9). Pressure on these points can be uncomfortable or painful. Do not work here for long; you will tire, and your partner will not benefit.

Chinese characters

Chinese characters are a visual representation of objects or ideas. You can see from the illustrations here how the characters for pressure point, or tsubo, and Channel describe the parts of their structure.

A tsubo

Roof

Skin surface

Thread or strand (communication)

Stream

Running water, underground

Work

Character for "Channel"

The Chinese were fond of using water as a metaphor for Ki. The Channels are like water courses and the points are like eddies, vortices, or swirls in the current. Like water, the Ki flows in the spaces between the muscles and other tissues of the body. These tissues are like the banks of a river: it is the water that creates the Channel, but the banks influence the flow.

The Path of Ki

The diagram below represents the movement of Ki in the body through successive pairs of Yin and Yang Channels. The flow of Ki is continuous but the cycle is traditionally described as beginning with the Lung Channel on the outer chest, as the Lungs are where Ki is formed. The sequence finishes with the Liver Channel, where Ki rejoins the Lung Channel and the cycle begins again. Each Yin Channel connects with its Yang counterpart on either the hand or the foot, where the change in polarity reverses the flow. The paired pathways occupy corresponding positions along the inner and outer aspects of the limbs. Yin channels join each other on the chest; Yang channels meet on the head or face. The diagram also shows the Yin–Yang Channels. The channels are paired: there is an above-below relationship as well as an inner-outer one. In the first group, Lung (Greater Yin) and Large Intestine (Sunrise Yang) on the arms are related to Stomach (Sunrise Yang) and Spleen (Greater Yin) on the legs. While each Yin–Yang pair belongs to the same Element (see p. 21), there is also a resonance between the Yin Channels and the Yang Channels of each quartet. They are like the upper and lower branches of the same Channel, whose shared traditional names suggest the complementary functions of their related organs and the similar Yin-Yang energy balance in each broad phase – morning, afternoon, and night. See "Chinese Clock" opposite.

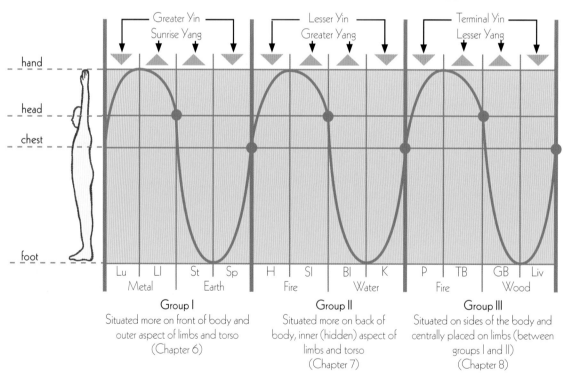

Group I	Group II	Group III
Situated more on front of body and outer aspect of limbs and torso (Chapter 6)	Situated more on back of body, inner (hidden) aspect of limbs and torso (Chapter 7)	Situated on sides of the body and centrally placed on limbs (between groups I and II) (Chapter 8)

Simplify your study and practice

Chapters 6, 7 and 8 deal with the paired Channels in these groups of four, explaining their relationship and demonstrating treatment routines for each group. Each chapter outlines a similar pattern.

To understand the body, and to understand health and disease, means going into detail. The various organs and their channels that you will study in the following chapters play distinct roles, but they work together, supporting each other as a systemic whole, as represented by the diagrams.

As you build on your knowledge and gain experience you will refine your skills, but you can keep your practice simple by following the above-below pattern as described when treating either the front, back or sides of the body, feeling for and learning to trust the subtle responses under your hands.

The continuing flow of Ki maintains harmony in the body by constantly adapting to the rhythms and demands of daily life as well as to abnormal stress and strain. There is naturally always some distortion. In our formal studies, "Yin and Yang" describes the basic pattern of the complementary forces involved, but our bodies will always respond positively to sensitive, simple touch. Shiatsu relies primarily on our experience of Nature. If we feel a resonance we can follow it.

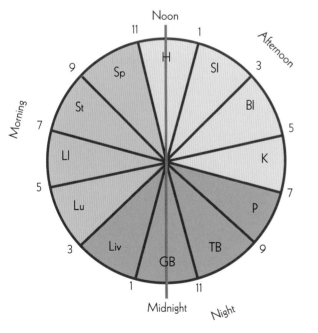

The "Chinese Clock"

According to tradition the activity of Ki intensifies in each Channel successively in a wave-like movement through the system, completing a cycle every 24 hours. Each Channel has a peak of activity lasting two hours and a correspondingly low phase 12 hours later. For example, the Bladder Channel is at its peak between three and five in the afternoon, and at its lowest phase between three and five in the morning. Observing the time of day when symptoms appear may indicate a disharmony of the relevant Channel. The model also highlights favoured times for certain exercises or activities in maintaining health.

The Yin and Yang Organs and their Channels

Traditional Oriental physiology and anatomy record a very different view of the body from that of modern Western medicine. The Yin and Yang Organs that form the core of the system are described in terms of their functions and interrelationships rather than their physical location, shape, structure, or chemistry. A significant example is the Triple Burner, an Organ in Chinese medicine, which has specific functions, harmonizing the upper, middle, and lower parts of the body, but has no physical counterpart (see also p. 125). Chinese medicine ascribes a much wider role to each of the Organs than does modern physiology, and their related Channels integrate the parts with the whole. Observation of patterns and connections, rather than analysis of component parts, has always been the way of Oriental medicine. Understanding their fundamental characteristics will help you recognize more easily which Organs are implicated in any illness, and the nature of the particular underlying imbalance.

Functions of the Yin Organs

There are five Yin Organs – the Lungs, Spleen, Heart, Kidneys, and Liver. Known as the "solid" Organs, they share the Yin characteristics of being internal, deep, and hidden. Yin Organs are the most important in the body; they are responsible for the transformation, circulation, and storage of Ki and Blood – pure substances essential to the body. Each of these Organs has Yin or Yang characteristics in varying degrees. Their functions are expressed in the quality and direction of movement of their Ki. Some are more concerned with Ki, some with Blood; some are situated higher in the body, some lower. The Lungs are on top, like a lid, and act downward. The Kidneys are at the bottom, and like roots, they hold and store Ki, but also send it upward. The Spleen also sends Ki up, while the Liver smooths and eases the flow of Ki whatever its direction.

Functions of the Yang Organs

The Yang Organs assist the Yin. Yang relates more to the surface or outside of things and generally the Yang or "hollow" Organs are those that make up the digestive tract (Gall Bladder, Stomach, Large Intestine, Small Intestine and Bladder). Defined only by their outer walls, they are concerned with receiving or processing food, or eliminating waste. In this sense they connect with the outside and their contents are unrefined – not yet usable by the body, or surplus to its needs. The Gall Bladder is the exception; it is a hollow Organ that stores a pure body fluid, bile, which helps digestion.

THE FUNCTIONS OF THE ORGANS AND
THE PATHWAYS OF KI AND BLOOD

The Lungs receive the air and transform the Ki of air and food into Human Ki. They disperse Ki to the skin for defence, circulate Ki in the Channels, and send surplus Ki down to be stored by the Kidneys.

The Liver stores Blood and eases all movements of Ki.

The Gall Bladder stores bile and assists the Liver.

The Stomach receives food and drink. It sends the purest parts to the Spleen and the less pure down to the Small Intestine. Stomach Ki goes down.

The Small Intestine separates and absorbs pure fluids and passes on impure fluids to the Bladder, and impure solids to the Large Intestine.

The Bladder stores and excretes the waste fluids.

The Large Intestine excretes the solid waste after absorbing fluids.

The "Triple Burner" has no location and no "form" but represents the whole system and its capacity to self-regulate and resist disease. It is thought of as acting throughout the body and integrating all its functions. See the distribution of Ki (p. 127).

The Pericardium – the outer muscle of the Heart – has its own Channel. As an Organ it assists and protects the Heart.

The Heart circulates Blood through all the vessels. It houses the Spirit.

The Spleen transforms and sends Ki and Essence of food up to Lungs. Essence is transformed into Blood. Food Ki is transformed into Human Ki.

The Kidneys send Ki up to the Spleen to activate the transformation of food, and to the Lungs to activate the transformation of Ki and Blood. The Kidneys store "Inherited Ki" or "Pre-natal Ki" as Essence, which is the basis of the constitution, affecting growth, maturity and reproduction. Kidney Ki is a mixture of Pre-natal Essence and Post-natal Ki. The Kidneys are the root and the foundation of Yin and Yang in the body.

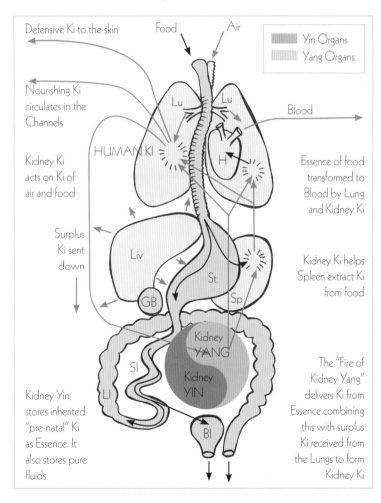

77

6. THE FRONT CHANNELS

LUNGS, LARGE INTESTINE, STOMACH, SPLEEN

This chapter, and the two that follow, each look at two pairs of Organs that are linked to each other in their work. They describe the functions of the related meridian pathways, or Channels (see pp. 80–81 and 84–85), illustrate exercises for each pair of Organs (see pp. 82–83 and 86–87), and end with a detailed routine for working on each group of Channels (see pp. 88–97).

The four Channels in this chapter are the first four in the cycle of Ki (see p. 74). As a group, these Channels deal with our need to absorb energy and sustenance from the environment after birth, and to discharge and return what is not required. Each of the Channels can be worked with your partner lying face up – the supine position.

The images and text on the facing page, and the corresponding sketches in the next two chapters, evoke archetypal bodily expressions of the quality of Ki in each pair of Organs and the primitive movement to the surface that the formal meridians represent. In this chapter, the Lungs and Large Intestine are the first pair of Organs (see top, facing page). They open to the outside and control the border between inside and out. The Lungs take energy in from the air and expel waste gases. They also control the skin, which "breathes".

The Large Intestine absorbs fluid and excretes solid wastes.

The second pair of Organs, the Stomach and Spleen, are the Organs of digestion (see bottom, facing page). Their Channels flow over the front of the body. The Spleen opens to the mouth and controls taste. The Stomach Channel passes from the eyes, around the mouth and through the centre of the breast. To the suckling infant, mouth, nipple, and warm embrace are all one thing. So begins our association of food and drink with security and comfort.

Once you have learned the pathways and tsubos in this chapter and the two that follow, you will have the basics from which to build your own routines. Remember to work with the principles and techniques described earlier in this book.

On being born, separate, alone in our own skin, the first breath comes with a cry, waking to new life. Each morning, waking to a new day. Stretch, open, and inhale deeply. Feel the outside space, fill the inside space. Then breathe out, relax, let go.

First and last; expanding; contractingl, opening; closing; defending the border

This is the full expression of the Lungs and Large Intestine.

The child reaches to its mother for sustenance and warmth. The mother reaches forward to hold and enfold the child. Later we must look further afield for our needs.

Become a hunter-gatherer, senses tuned; seek special information, learn discrimination. Shopping, or picking wild fruits and herbs; studying, or reaching out for contact.

Stomach and Spleen Ki always moves to the front.

The Lung Channel pathway

The Lung Channel begins deep in the solar plexus region (the Middle Burner, see p. 127) and descends to meet the Large Intestine, the Yang Organ paired with the Lungs. Winding up past the Stomach, it crosses the diaphragm, divides, and enters the Lungs. It then re-unites, passes up the middle of the windpipe to the throat and divides again, surfacing in the hollow region near the front of the shoulder (Lu 1).

From here it passes over the shoulder and down the anterior (front) aspect of the arm along the outer border of the biceps muscle.

It reaches the outside of the biceps tendon in the elbow crease (Lu 5), and continues down the forearm to the wrist just above the base of the thumb (Lu 9). The Channel crosses the height of the thumb muscle to finish at the corner of the thumbnail.

The Lung Channel – functions and symptoms

The Lungs rule Ki. They receive, transform, and distribute it in the body; to the skin for defence, through the Channels to nourish and energize all parts, and down to all the other Organs, especially the Kidneys, where surplus post-natal Ki adds to our constitutional reserves.

If the Lungs are weak they cannot supply enough Ki to the skin for defence; climatic influences can then invade through the pores. This according to Oriental medicine is how we "catch" chills, colds, fevers, and stiff neck from sitting in a draught. A chronic weakness of the Lungs generally produces tiredness, often breathlessness, and a pale complexion. If the Lungs cannot circulate Ki, it accumulates, producing a tight, stuffy chest and a cough,

or asthma. Other Lung symptoms may need treatment on more than one Channel; for example, a dry, irritating cough, dry throat, and dry skin often require work on the Kidney Channel as well.

Channel symptoms

Pain and other symptoms occurring along the superficial course of a Channel are called "Channel symptoms". They will benefit from work on the Channel. In the Lung Channel these include chest and shoulder pains, pain along the arm or in the thumb, and stiff neck.

THE LUNG CHANNEL Arm Greater Yin

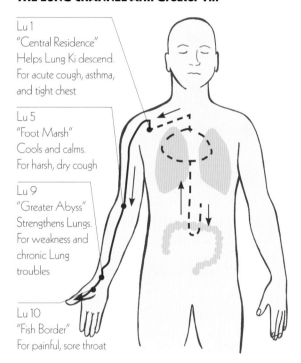

Lu 1
"Central Residence"
Helps Lung Ki descend.
For acute cough, asthma,
and tight chest

Lu 5
"Foot Marsh"
Cools and calms.
For harsh, dry cough

Lu 9
"Greater Abyss"
Strengthens Lungs.
For weakness and
chronic Lung
troubles

Lu 10
"Fish Border"
For painful, sore throat

Internal pathway symptoms

For throat problems, loss of voice, asthma, breathlessness, bronchitis, bowel problems – constipation, colitis, etc.

The Large Intestine Channel pathway

The Large Intestine Channel begins by the outside corner of the index fingernail. It runs along the edge of the finger, between the two tendons of the thumb at the wrist joint (LI 5) and along the bony margin of the outer edge of the arm (the radius bone) to the elbow. The point LI 11 is situated at the outside of the elbow crease, which is visible when the arm is bent. From here the Channel continues to the point LI 15 on the outside of the shoulder muscle. It then crosses the shoulder blade and meets the Governing Vessel below the 7th cervical vertebra at point GV 14. It descends internally to connect first with the Lung and then with its own Organ, the Large Intestine. From the shoulder a branch travels upward over the muscle at the side of the neck (sterno-cleido-mastoid) to the cheek, passing through the lower gums, then round over the top lip. It terminates beside the opposite nostril, where it links to the Stomach Channel.

Large Intestine – functions and symptoms

The Large Intestine receives the remaining part of food and drink from the Small Intestine, absorbs more fluids, and excretes the residue. It can be unbalanced by improper diet, acute illness, weakness, or worry, although these are often better treated indirectly through a related Channel, rather than by the Large Intestine Channel itself.

For example, many bowel troubles will respond better to treatment of the Lung, Kidney, Spleen, or Stomach Channels. For problems created by worry, or constipation associated with weakness or breathlessness,

treat the Lungs. Weak or chilly people are often prone to watery stools of diarrhoea, with rumblings, distension, and abdominal discomfort. In this case treat the Spleen, which controls transformation of fluids.

Treat the Large Intestine Channel for shoulder pain and tennis elbow, and blockages or pain in the sensory organs, including nasal congestion, sinusitis, or toothache. Work on this Channel from elbow to hand for constipation that is due to heat or fever.

THE LARGE INTESTINE CHANNEL
Arm Sunrise Yang

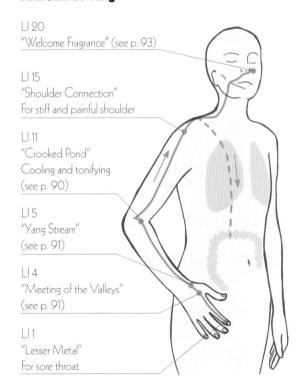

LI 20
"Welcome Fragrance" (see p. 93)

LI 15
"Shoulder Connection"
For stiff and painful shoulder

LI 11
"Crooked Pond"
Cooling and tonifying
(see p. 90)

LI 5
"Yang Stream"
(see p. 91)

LI 4
"Meeting of the Valleys"
(see p. 91)

LI 1
"Lesser Metal"
For sore throat

Internal pathway symptoms

For constipation in acute illness and fevers or due to weak Lungs

CHANNEL EXERCISES
LUNGS & LARGE INTESTINE

The Oriental tradition of doing exercises for longevity and health includes some that strengthen particular Organs and improve the flow of Ki in the Channels. A few such exercises are given below for the Lungs and Large Intestine.

A common thread in all traditional exercises is the importance attached to the breath. Good breathing is the source of our vitality. The Lungs govern respiration, rule Ki, and open into the nose. The Large Intestine Channel finishes at the nose and helps regulate breathing. Nowadays people suffer greatly from obstructed nasal passages, allergic rhinitis, and general problems from polluted city air and air "conditioning".

Refined, processed and de-natured foods weaken the Large Intestine and are often linked with allergies, and both Lung and Large Intestine are affected by worry and stress, and the effects of sedentary living. Walking, swimming, cycling, and hill climbing, as well as formal exercises and deep nasal breathing, counter many of these negative influences.

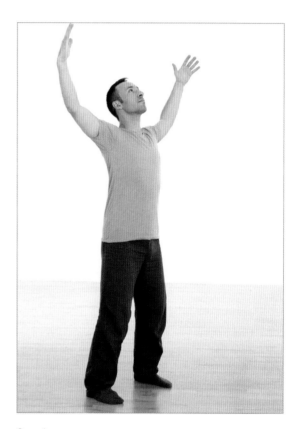

Stretching

Yawning boosts the oxygen in the Blood. To induce a yawn, rub your face next to your mouth and nose, then stretch and open your mouth. We can make this spontaneous stretching into a formal exercise. Breathe in as you raise your arms, then circle them round, looking upward. Pause for a moment with your arms stretched back (see above). Feel the Ki flow along the Channels. Exhale as you lower your arms.

Makko Ho stretches

Masunaga adopted a series of stretches for each pair of Channels from the Japanese exercise system known as Makko Ho. These have become widely associated with shiatsu – good for givers and receivers alike. They are all based on the spontaneous expressions – the natural movement of Ki in daily life that corresponds with each meridian pair.

Lung and Large Intestine Makko Ho

For the Lungs and Large Intestine, stand with your feet apart. Link your thumbs behind you, then exhale and bend forward from your hips, stretching your arms out and up, knees slightly bent (see right). Breathe and relax further into it for a few breaths. Uncurl slowly as you exhale.

The Stomach Channel path way

Starting beside the nose, near LI 20, the Stomach Channel meets the Bladder Channel at Point Bl 1 on the forehead. From St 1, just below the eye, it passes into the upper gums and round the mouth to link with the Governing and Directing Vessels. Next, via the lower gums, it ascends in front of the ear to the forehead.

From the jaw it descends alongside the throat to the collarbone region, where an internal branch descends to meet the Stomach and Spleen. The superficial path continues down over the abdomen to the pubic area, where a second internal branch from the Stomach rejoins it.

The Channel continues down the anterior thigh, passing just to the outside of the kneecap. At St 36, below the knee, the Channel divides again. The surface branch runs down the leg beside the shinbone, ending on the outside of the second toe. The deeper branch descends to the middle toe. From the top of the foot a connection runs to the Spleen Channel.

The Stomach and Spleen in digestion

The Stomach and Spleen share the role of digestion and are often considered and treated together. Ki from food is the basis of the body's Ki and Blood, so it is important to strengthen both Stomach and Spleen in any chronic illness.

The Stomach suffers most from dryness and heat. It "likes wetness and dislikes dryness". If its fluids are deficient, digestion will suffer and the mouth and lips will become dry. The Stomach directs Ki downward. If disturbed the Ki may "rebel" upward causing nausea, vomiting, or headaches.

THE STOMACH CHANNEL Leg Sunrise Yang

St 1
"Containing Tears"
(see p. 92)

St 3
"Big Bone"

St 8
"Head Support"
For headaches, muzzy, heavy head, dizziness, eye troubles (see p. 92)

St 34
"Beam Mound"
For acute stomach trouble, mastitis

St 36
"Leg Three Miles"
(see p. 94)

St 44
"Inner Courtyard"
(see p. 95)

Internal pathway symptoms

Teeth and gum troubles, indigestion, nausea and vomiting

THE SPLEEN CHANNEL Leg Greater Yin

Connects with Lung Channel (Lu 1)

Sp 10
"Sea of Blood"
(see p. 97)

Sp 9
"Yin Mountain Pond" (see p. 97)

Sp 6
"Three-Yin Meeting"
(see p. 97)

Sp 3
"Greater Whiteness"
(see p. 97)

Internal pathway symptoms

Weak digestion, inability to taste foods, flat or dirty taste in mouth. Menstrual and reproductive organ problems

The Spleen Channel pathway

Beginning on the inside tip of the big toe, the Spleen Channel follows the inner aspect of the foot to the arch, then turns up in front of the inner ankle to Sp 6. It continues up the leg, just behind the bone, crossing the knee and ascending the anterior thigh from the inner border of the kneecap.

From the groin it enters the lower abdomen, meets the Directing Vessel, then resurfaces briefly before penetrating the Spleen and Stomach. The main Channel then ascends through the diaphragm, over the chest, and crosses the Lung Channel at Lu 1. It continues up to the oesophagus and under the tongue. An inner branch from the Stomach region transports Ki up to the Heart.

The functions of the Spleen

The principal role of the Spleen is transforming and transporting. It transforms food and conveys the nourishing Ki to the Organs, muscles, and limbs and up to the Heart and Lungs as the basis for Ki and Blood. Its warming Yang Ki also transforms body fluids. The Spleen likes dryness, and hates damp. Cold foods or too many cold drinks can weaken the Spleen. Symptoms are poor appetite and digestion, tiredness, weak muscles, heavy limbs, watery stools or diarrhoea, and swollen abdomen.

Spleen Ki also "holds the Blood", preventing haemorrhage, and "holds up" the Organs. Bruising, bleeding, haemorrhoids, varicose veins, and all forms of prolapse are symptoms of Spleen weakness.

CHANNEL EXERCISES
STOMACH & SPLEEN

The following exercises help harmonize the Stomach and Spleen. Their Channels flow over the front of the body. The Spleen houses the intellect. Too much intellectual work or studying, especially when associated with irregular eating habits, can weaken the Spleen. In the same way, inability to concentrate, or poor memory, are symptoms of depleted Spleen. Exercise forms the ideal balance to intellectual work.

The sense of taste in the Five Element system is associated with the Spleen (see p. 21). The inability to taste food, or a dull, flat taste in the mouth indicate a Stomach–Spleen disharmony, as does craving for sweet foods – the specific flavour of the Earth Organs.

Stomach and Spleen Makko Ho stretch

From the seiza position (see p. 30), sit as low as you can between your heels. Do not proceed if your knees are painful but practise "just sitting" until you are comfortable. Lean back on your hands, lifting and opening your chest. Then drop on to your elbows (see above) and finally all the way down. Stretch your arms over your head if it is comfortable. Exhale as you move into each new position. Breathe 3 times in your final stretch. Move back through every stage slowly.

The Camel Pose

This yoga posture is an alternative stretch for people whose knees will not permit the stronger Makko Ho stretch. You can start this from an easy position, even sitting on a cushion between your heels. Kneel up and bring your hands on to your heels to support your body. Lift your pelvis up and forward to arch your body on a full exhalation. Hold for a few breaths before coming out of the position.

Stress and tension in the jaw

You may not think of the face as needing exercise, but it does. Stress and tension, often held unconsciously in the jaw muscle, may result in clenching and teeth grinding at night – a common problem.

Jaw stretching

The best exercise is to chew your food well, which benefits the Stomach directly. But you can also stretch, grimace, and move your jaw, and vocalize your feelings too. A more subtle, traditional exercise is to run your tongue around your gums to generate saliva — considered a precious fluid associated with the Spleen. Swallow and relax.

Tension in the diaphragm and stomach

The diaphragm, the stomach, and the solar plexus area are often held in tension, inhibiting breathing and circulation of Ki and Blood to the digestive Organs.

Releasing the solar plexus

With your fingers turned in to the area just below your ribcage, lean forward to apply gradually increasing pressure (see right). Always exhale slowly as you lean forward. Inhale as you sit up. Repeat a few times. The effect is purifying and invigorating.

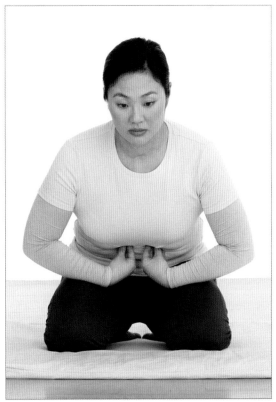

SHIATSU ROUTINE FOR THE FRONT CHANNELS

You can reach the Lung, Large Intestine, Stomach, and Spleen Channels most easily with your partner lying face up (the supine position). Work on the Lung and Spleen Channels strengthens Ki and aids its circulation around the body. It warms the limbs and strengthens digestion. Bear in mind their specific functions (see pp. 80 and 85) as you give shiatsu along these Channels.

The Large Intestine and Stomach Channels (see pp. 81 and 84) meet on the face. Work on them can help in troubles of the eyes, nose, sinuses, teeth, and gums. The routine that follows on pages 89–101 starts with the arms, continues with the head and neck, and finishes on the legs.

Quiet preparation

Relax in seiza position by your partner's side and make contact by resting your palm on their Hara. Calm and centre yourself by taking note of how you feel and by acknowledging your condition. Pay attention to your partner's breathing. This is particularly important for your work on the Lung Channel.

Stay relaxed

Remember, keep your shoulders relaxed, extend your arms, and lean from your Hara. Don't squeeze or press with your thumb – it won't be effective and it may hurt.

Lung

Spleen

Treat them as one meridian "Greater Yin"

Large Intestine

Stomach

One channel, one path "Sunrise Yang"

Simplify theory and practice

1. Initial arm rotation

Pick up your partner's arm with your outside hand and move your other hand from the Hara to clasp the top of your partner's shoulder. Lift the arm over your partner's head, then bring it round and down, out to the side. Repeat a few times (see p. 48), then place it on the floor at an angle of 45 degrees to your partner's side.

2. Lung Channel position

In order to lean comfortably and contact the Ki of the Lung Channel, move to the outside of the arm, facing in, with your partner's palm facing upward. Support your partner's shoulder with your nearside hand. Now lean into the hollow area at the front of the shoulder (corresponding to points Lu 1 and Lu 2) and place your other hand anywhere along the arm (see above). Pause and relax, knees spread wide, before palming down the Channel.

3. Palming the Lung Channel

With your active hand locate the biceps muscle, and lean your weight through the line of your extended thumb and the heel of your palm into the space between the muscle and the humerus bone. Ease up, slide your hand along an inch or two, then relax and repeat the pressure. Continue in this way on the near side of the arm, palming down in easy stages to the wrist on the thumb side. Finish by gently squeezing along the sides of the thumb (see above).

4. Thumbing the Lung Channel (investigating the groove)

Now, with your fingers supporting the arm, use your extended thumb to explore the groove between the biceps muscle and the bone, for the tsubos. Slide your thumb along between these points, always keeping contact. Work into Lu 5 (see p. 80) on the outside of the biceps tendon at the elbow. Continue thumbing down the Channel, just inside the radius bone, toward Lu 9 at the base of the thumb (see p. 80). Pause to lean into the tsubos you find along the way.

5. Thumbing the thumb at Lu 10

Finish by grasping the base of your partner's thumb and squeezing firmly along its edges to the corners of the nail. Alternatively, thumb along the inside edge, including the "belly" of the muscle at the base of the thumb, where Lu 10 is found. This is a sedating point for painful sore throats.

The Large Intestine Channel

You can work on this Channel with very little adjustment to your position. All you need to do is rotate your partner's hand slightly inward to bring the edge of the forearm uppermost. The Large Intestine Channel runs close to the Lung Channel, but as it is Yang it is nearer to the outside of the arm, along the bony edge.

6. Palming the Large Intestine Channel

Lean on the outer part of your partner's shoulder with your support hand. Then gently grasp the upper arm with the other hand, and feel for the LI Channel along the humerus bone (see above). Work with your flattened thumb and heel of your palm. Move your hand down in stages past the elbow, leaning and gently grasping, then along the bony edge of the forearm.

7. Thumbing the Large Intestine Channel

When you are familiar with the location of this Channel, try using your thumb at a more penetrating angle to work the upper arm (see above). Work down to LI 11, at the outside end of the elbow crease when the arm is folded. Use this point for feverish and hot conditions, rashes and itching. Below the elbow use the "Dragon's Mouth" technique (see p. 44) to work down in stages from the elbow to the wrist.

Large Intestine 4

Find the high point of the muscle between the forefinger and thumb when closed. As your partner relaxes the muscle, press firmly down and toward the finger bone. This widely used point relieves aches and pains of the head, jaw, and teeth. It strengthens Yang and defensive Ki, and expels Wind, Cold, and Heat symptoms from the face, such as streaming colds, sneezing, sore eyes, and hay fever. Internally it has a strong downward action that helps constipation and childbirth.

Caution: Do not use this point during pregnancy.

8. Thumbing on the hand

At the wrist joint use your thumb to give pressure to LI 5, located between the two tendons of the thumb. It is useful for pain in the wrist or thumb.

The LI Channel finishes on the forefinger. Grip or thumb along its edge to the nail and then pause for a moment when you finish, before quietly breaking contact and moving round to work on the Lung and LI Channels on the other side.

Leaning on the shoulders at Lung 1. After working along the Large Intestine and Lung channels you can help integrate the effects by gently leaning into the hollows just below the shoulders (Lu 1). Bring your weight forward gently with steady pressure, holding a short time while giving space to your partner's breath. This point "moves Ki down", helps deepen the breathing and relieves sensations of tightness and heaviness in the chest.

Working on the face and neck

Pause after finishing the arms, then keeping a light contact at your partner's shoulder if you can, move to a kneeling position with your knees spread wide either side of your partner's ears. Do not kneel too close as this will restrict your working circle, and may feel oppressive to your partner. Work on this area requires sensitivity. Approach the head and neck in a relaxed state of mind. Lean with both hands on your partner's shoulders and relax.

Loosening the neck

Rest the palms of your hands loosely over the temples and ears for a few moments then, with your fingertips, hold the occipital ridge at the base of the skull behind the ears. Roll the head gently a few times from side to side to loosen the neck. Then, resting the edges of your hands on the floor, move your fingers farther under the head and curl them back into the hollows beneath the occipital bone. Lean back from the Hara to open and stretch the neck. This raises the back of your partner's head off the floor. Then slide your palms underneath so that the head rests comfortably in your hands. Keep your fingers where they are, cupping the back of the head – a pleasant sensation for your partner. Pause for a moment or two.

9. Working the Stomach Channel on the face and neck

Roll your partner's head to the side, cradling and balancing it on the open palm and fingers of one hand. The other hand is now free to work the Stomach Channel along both its branches (see above) with the extended thumb. Begin at the point just inside the hairline at the corner of the forehead, St 8. The Channel passes down the side of the head, about 1 in (2.5 cm) in front of the ear. Feel for tsubos, including St 7 under the cheek bone and St 6 near the angle of the jaw in the middle of the powerful chewing muscle (Masseter muscle).

The other branch of this Channel begins on the border of the eye socket (the orbit) at St 1 and St 2. St 3 is under the cheek bone, level with the widest part of the nose. This point is good for sneezing and nasal troubles.

10. LI 20 "Welcome Fragrance"

"Welcome Fragrance" is the last point of the LI Channel. As the name suggests, stimulating this point will help clear a sore, stuffy nose or sinuses. You may feel that your index finger or even your little finger is better suited to stimulating LI 20. Extend the finger and lean at a slight angle upward and in toward the nose using the weight of your relaxed arm (see above).

12. Lifting the neck and stretching the spine

Return your partner's head to its natural position, move your hands down and overlap your fingers to encircle the underside of the neck below the skull. Keep your thumbs tucked positively against your partner's jawbone. Lift up and back, gently arching the neck and, by sinking back from your hips, give a little stretch to the spine. Replace the head on the ground, pulling back slightly on the occipital ridge under the skull. Finish the routine as you began, leaning on your partner's shoulders. Gently break contact after a few moments.

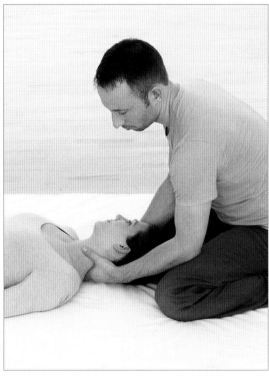

11. Working the neck

Still cradling the head at a slight angle (see above), work down the prominent muscle at the side of the neck (sterno-cleido-mastoid). The LI Channel runs along its top, and the Stomach Channel a little to the front. Rest the ball of your thumb over the muscle, the fingers of your working hand supporting the back of your partner's neck. Try to feel as if your two hands are cooperating and connected (see p. 50). Alter the attitude of your partner's head a little to promote relaxation as you work down both Channels on the muscle.

Work on the other side

Replace the working hand under the skull to match the position of the other one, before rolling the head over gently to repeat the work on Stomach and Large Intestine Channels on the other side of the face.

Positioning for the Leg Channels

The Stomach and Spleen Channels descend the front of the thigh and leg. The Stomach Channel, being Yang, runs outside the Yin Spleen Channel (see p. 85). The Stomach and Spleen govern digestion and belong to the Earth Element. Work on their Channels in the leg will connect your partner "energetically" with the Earth (see p. 20) and strengthen digestion. Kneel facing your partner, your knees spread wide.

13. Palming the Stomach Channel

Place one hand below the navel; the other, fingers pointing out, on top of your partner's thigh. Palm down in stages to the knee, turning your fingers inward once you are below the level of the groin. Then try the Stomach Channel stretch (below left).

14. Stretching the Stomach Channel

Roll your partner's near leg inward and extend your own leg to rest the sole of your foot, heel on the ground, across the front of your partner's foot. This brings the Stomach Channel uppermost. Then kneel up, bring your hips forward, and palm the Channel again, this time from the upper thigh to the lower leg. The stretch activates the Ki in the Channel. It may seem difficult, but try it.

15. Thumbing the Stomach Channel

From the same position thumb the Stomach Channel down the leg. Slide your thumb between tsubos to St 34, 2 in (5 cm) above the kneecap. Continue over the knee to St 36 — one hand's breadth below the kneecap (see above), and down the leg, following the Stomach Channel about one finger-width outside the shinbone.

16. Thumbing the Stomach Channel on the foot

As you reach the foot, bring your supporting hand down from the Hara to any part of the leg, above or below the knee, or even to the ankle. Thumb over the highest part of the foot (see above) to St 44 between the 2nd and 3rd toes (see right). Work into St 44, then to the end of the Channel on the outside of the second toe; squeeze it firmly and stretch it.

St 44

Stomach 36 ("Leg Three Miles")

Ancient physicians said that any disease could be treated by this point. It can be used to strengthen and tonify the whole system safely. St 36 works on the Stomach and the Spleen, which according to traditional Oriental medicine extract Blood and Ki from food. It is said that Chinese foot soldiers used to halt every three miles and massage St 36 for renewed energy – hence its name. Soldiers of the revolutionary peasant army who followed Mao Tse Tung on the incredible "Long March" across China, 1934–35, are reported to have done the same.

Stomach 44 ("Inner Courtyard")

Half an inch (1cm) before the web between the second and third toes is St 44. To find this point press toward the bone of the second toe. Work on St 44 to alleviate stomach ache or acidity; for acute problems work on St 36 and St 34 as well. St 44 will also help relieve toothache, sore or bleeding gums, redness and irritation of the eyes, or frontal headaches. For problems of the face or mouth also work on the Large Intestine Channel, especially LI 4 (see p. 81).

The Spleen Channel

Work on the Spleen Channel can help with all problems of the joints in the leg, hip, knee, ankle, and big toe. It is especially useful when pain is felt on the path of the Spleen Channel and if it feels worse in damp weather. Both dampness and the Spleen are associated with the Earth element (see p. 20 and Chapter 9). The Spleen also helps with the transformation and movement of fluids within the body. Feelings of heaviness or bloating in the abdomen and legs, or fluid around the ankles (oedema), for example, can also be treated by working on this Channel. The Spleen controls Blood, helping to produce it, and keeping it within the vessels. In women, menstrual problems such as scanty or missing periods, or bleeding in between periods, may respond to work on the Spleen Channel. More generally, frequent nose-bleeds, bleeding piles, easy bruising, and mild varicose veins are conditions related to the Spleen. Finally, some troubles of the lower digestive tract, especially diarrhoea, can benefit from work on this Channel.

Caution: Do not give shiatsu on the Spleen Channel during pregnancy if miscarriage is likely. Do not use Sp 6 during any pregnancy.

17. Rotating the leg

Keep one hand on the Hara and reach around under the knee with the other. Lean forward to lift and bend the knee. With your partner's foot still on the ground, rest the leg against your side. Bring your hand out to push up on the front of the knee (see above) and rotate the leg in a controlled way, using your body weight. Rotate the hip inward and forward, around, out, and back a few times.

18. Starting work on the Spleen Channel

After the rotations place your partner's leg down, tucked against your body. Lift the ankle and slide the toes to the ankle of the other leg (see above). Let your partner's knee fall gently outward. This brings the Spleen Channel uppermost.

19. Palming the Spleen Channel

Kneeling up and forward, support your partner's knee on your thigh. Lean on to your partner's inner thigh. Palm the Spleen Channel past the inner edge of the kneecap to ankle, turning your fingers inward as you go down the thigh (see p. 60).

20. Thumbing the Spleen Channel

After palming, the tsubos on the Spleen Channel will be easier to find. The classical points, Sp 10, 9, 6 and 3, described below, are useful to know and act as landmarks on the way. Slide your thumb lightly along the Channel, working into receptive points. The inner leg can be tender: move from your Hara to increase pressure gradually (see p. 51).

Spleen 3 ("Greater Whiteness")

This point is just behind the prominent joint of the big toe on the side of the foot, slightly beneath the bone (see below). Its name suggests a pallid complexion associated with weak Blood. Spleen 3 strengthens the Spleen and helps when weak digestion is combined with poor appetite, when bowel motions are loose, or if there is colonic bleeding. This point helps poor memory, muddled thinking, or mental fatigue. It also strengthens the neck and spine.

Spleen 3

Spleen 6 ("Three-Yin Meeting")

Spleen 6 is found one hand's breadth up from the inside ankle bone, in the hollow in the muscle just behind the bone. The three Yin Channels of the Spleen, Liver, and Kidneys meet here. Generally, Sp 6 strengthens and regulates Blood. It is used in all male and female sexual problems – impotence, infertility, menstrual irregularities, period pains, and discharges. In women it influences the uterus, promoting contractions during childbirth and easing labour pains (see Chapter 10).
Caution: Do not use SP 6 during pregnancy.

Spleen 9 ("Yin Mountain Pond")

This point is about 2 in (5 cm) below the knee on the inside, in the hollow between the head of the large bone (the tibia) and the calf muscle. It helps the Spleen to control fluids and is useful for pains in the knee, especially those made worse by damp, and when stiffness increases with lack of movement, for example, in bed or sitting still.

Spleen 10 ("Sea of Blood")

Just 2 in (5 cm) above the kneecap on its inner edge, in the height of the muscular bulge, is Sp 10. The point is useful to control bleeding in people who have a tendency toward mild haemorrhages. It has a cooling action on the Blood and will ease hot rashes and itching.

7. THE BACK CHANNELS

HEART, SMALL INTESTINE, BLADDER, KIDNEY

The Heart, deep and hidden, is the Organ of central control, the seat of consciousness and "House of the Mind"; the centre of response to the emotional environment. It governs Blood and controls blood vessels and circulation. Blood not only nourishes the physical body but embraces and supports the Mind. Like the emperor of old, performing sacred rites to harmonize the elements and ensure peace and prosperity among the people, when the Heart performs well the body flourishes and the Mind is serene and happy. Those people who have a strong constitution, a lively mind, a sparkle in their eyes, and an open, warm, and sensible disposition reflect the work of this Organ. The Small Intestine absorbs nutrients from food to enrich the blood. It assists the Heart by clarifying our thoughts, and absorbing the effects of shock. The archetypal expression for these meridians is that of serenity, inner composure.

The heart channel, on the folded inner arms' surface, is appropriately hidden.

The Kidneys are equally fundamental. They are called the "Root of Life". All organisms are impelled by the need to survive; to protect themselves and reproduce. The impetus of these drives manifests through the Kidneys. Assisted by the Bladder, they control purification, energy reserves, efficient hormonal and nervous systems, preparedness, and power to take action. The Kidneys are the foundation of Yin and Yang. They store constitutional Essence, and govern birth, growth, and reproduction.

In Five Element terms, Heart and Small Intestine (see top, facing page) belong to Fire, the uprising tendency, summer, heat, the colour red, the sound of laughter, and the emotion of joy or happiness. By contrast the Bladder and Kidneys (see bottom, facing page) belong to Water, the sinking, collecting tendency, winter, cold, the colour blue-black, the groaning sound, and the emotion of fear. Their Channels follow the inner and back surface of the legs and are closely parallel to the spine and mid line Channels. The archetypal image here is "prepare to run" – to escape danger, or to attain a goal. You can work on all four Channels with your partner lying face down – the prone position.

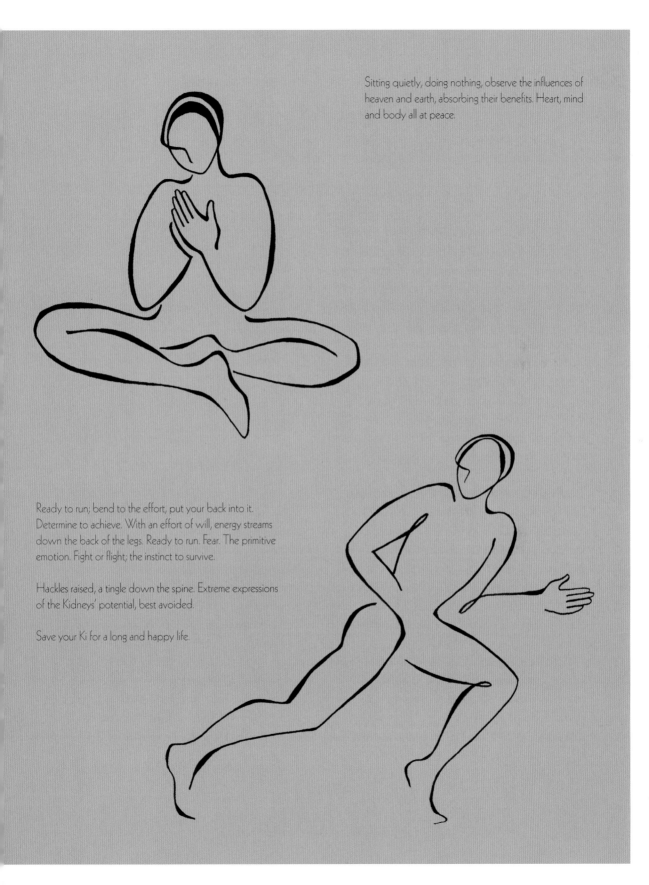

Sitting quietly, doing nothing, observe the influences of heaven and earth, absorbing their benefits. Heart, mind and body all at peace.

Ready to run; bend to the effort, put your back into it. Determine to achieve. With an effort of will, energy streams down the back of the legs. Ready to run. Fear. The primitive emotion. Fight or flight; the instinct to survive.

Hackles raised, a tingle down the spine. Extreme expressions of the Kidneys' potential, best avoided.

Save your Ki for a long and happy life.

The Heart Channel pathway

This Channel begins in the Heart and emerges via the surrounding blood vessels to pass down through the diaphragm to the Small Intestine, its related Organ. Another internal branch ascends through the throat to the eye, and a connecting Channel goes to the tongue.

A third branch goes first to the Lung before surfacing at the centre of the armpit. From here the Channel descends along the inner aspect of the arm, on the opposite side of the biceps to the Lung Channel, passing the inner end of the elbow crease. It continues down to the tip of the little finger by the corner of the nail on the thumb side.

When giving shiatsu in the supine position it is best to fold the arm into the Heart Channel stretch position (see right), which makes it easily accessible. For shiatsu in the prone position, as in this chapter, work with the arm away from the side, palm turned up.

The Heart Channel – functions and symptoms

Constitutional strength depends on the Heart as well as the Kidneys (see p. 105). Accordingly, disorders of the Heart may result in weakness, tiredness, or lethargy, and sometimes in dizziness or palpitations. The close relationship of Blood and Ki means that the Lungs may be affected as well, resulting in breathlessness (see p. 80).

The Heart belongs to the Fire element, moves Blood, and houses the Mind. The Channel opens to the tongue and controls sweat. Heart disharmonies are often characterized by disorders of the circulation, such as stuffiness or pains in the chest, and feeling too hot or too

THE HEART CHANNEL
Arm Lesser Yin

H 7
"Mind Door"

H 3
"Lesser Yin Sea"
Cooling and mentally
calming

H 1
"Supreme Spring"

H 7
"Mind Door"
Calms the mind;
relaxing, easing

H 9
"Lesser Yin Rushing"
Stimulates Heart.
For stroke or heart attack

Internal pathway symptoms
For stammering, incoherent speech, heart problems

cold, especially in the hands. Imbalance in the Heart may also produce mental and emotional disorders such as restlessness, insomnia, or dream-disturbed sleep, and nervousness, irritability, or anxiety. Abnormal sweating may accompany any of these symptoms.

The face colour reflects the state of the circulation and, therefore, of the Heart (see pp. 156–7). A pale, lifeless complexion suggests weakness of Heart Ki or Blood; a red complexion indicates that Heat is affecting the Heart. Heart disharmonies show themselves in the tongue, producing speech difficulties, such as stammering.

The Small Intestine Channel pathway

This Channel starts on the other corner of the little fingernail from the Heart Channel (see facing page) and follows the edge of the hand to the wrist, where it turns slightly to flow up the forearm, close to the outer edge of the (ulna) bone. Passing the elbow at the "funny bone", it continues up the back of the arm, behind the shoulder joint. It then curves across the shoulder blade to connect with the Governing Vessel at GV 14 as do all Yang Channels. It crosses forward to the hollow above the collarbone where the internal branch penetrates, first to the Heart, then along the oesophagus to the Stomach, before connecting with its own Organ, the Small Intestine.

From the collarbone region the superficial path continues up behind the muscle on the side of the neck (sterno-cleido-mastoid), then over the cheek to the ear. Two internal branches separate on the cheek. They lead to the Gall Bladder Channel on the outer corner of the eye, and to the Bladder Channel – the next in the cycle (see p. 75) – at Bl 1 on the inner corner.

The Small Intestine – functions and symptoms

The Small Intestine receives partially transformed food and drink from the Stomach and separates and absorbs the nourishing part for the Spleen to distribute. It moves the solid waste to the Large Intestine, passing "impure fluids" to the Bladder. The role of this Channel can be summarized as receiving, separating, assimilating, and transforming. The Small Intestine is linked with the Heart, and helps it to give clarity to the Mind, discerning and absorbing good ideas. Muddled thinking is a

THE SMALL INTESTINE CHANNEL
Arm Greater Yang

SI 19
"Listening Palace"
For ear problems

SI 18
"Cheek Bone"

Shoulder points
(see p. 109)

SI 6
"Nourishing the Old"
For tightness and stiffness of neck, shoulders, and low back

SI 3 "Back Stream"
(see p. 112)

Internal pathway symptoms

For styes, sore eyes, loose stools sometimes with scant, burning urination

sign of weakness in the Small Intestine.

The role of separating and transforming fluids is shared with the Bladder. Both Organs are located in the lower region of the body, controlled by the Kidneys. Because of the Bladder connections, work on the Small Intestine Channel helps to relieve posterior headaches and pain in the spine and lower back. Frequent and profuse, or scanty, burning urination may be treated by work on these three Channels. Channel symptoms of the Small Intestine include pain and stiffness of the wrist, elbow, or shoulder blade area and neck, earache, and sore, red eyes.

CHANNEL EXERCISES
HEART & SMALL INTESTINE

Stress, poor diet, and over-eating are now recognized as the main causes of circulation and heart troubles. If you are too rushed to choose foods wisely and too stressed to eat and digest comfortably, you will weaken your constitution and jeopardize your heart.

The Heart Channel goes to the tongue and helps the Spleen to distinguish the "five flavours" and so choose appropriate foods. The Small Intestine supports the Stomach and Spleen in digestion, as well as assisting your judgement in all matters.

The Heart and Small Intestine Makko Ho exercise derives from the posture of prayer and meditation. The stretch gently activates both Channels by opening the neck and shoulders, which stimulates the course of Ki in the Channels in the arm. It also opens and invigorates the chest and abdominal cavities where the Organs are located. The simple message behind these exercises is – eat less and relax more.

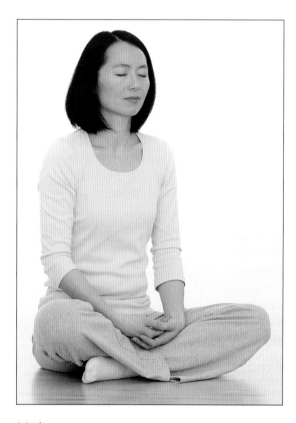

Meditation pose

It is not so much the formal posture that is important — more the inner practice. Sit or kneel in any position with your spine relaxed and upright. Use a cushion or sit in a chair if you like. Relax your hands, close your eyes, and spend up to 15 minutes just being aware of your breath or listening to its sound. You will be distracted, but do not worry; just start again. There is nothing to achieve; nowhere to go.

Empty the Heart of everything, let the Mind be at peace.

TAO TE CHING, LAO TZU

Heart and Small Intestine Makko Ho stretch

Sit with your knees bent and the soles of your feet together. Clasp your feet, bringing them as close to your groin as comfortable. Let your knees drop. Then, using your feet as an anchor, lift open your chest and exhaling slowly, fold forward from this position until the end of the breath. Relax in the furthest position, elbows outside the knees, breathing several times into your Hara. Inhale as you sit up.

The Bladder Channel pathway

The Bladder Channel begins at the inner corner of the eye, rising up through the eyebrow (Bl 2) over the forehead and skull to join the Governing Vessel at GV 20. Here it enters the brain, re-emerging as a superficial path at the nape of the neck. This path continues over the base of the skull (occiput), where it divides again into two branches that descend parallel with the spine. The inner branch diverts briefly to meet GV 14 before continuing to the sacrum, then on down the back of the thigh to the centre of the kneefold. An internal branch connects with the Kidney and then the Bladder, after separating at the lumbar region. The outer branch passes from the occiput along the edge of the shoulder blade and descends to the buttock, continuing down the thigh to meet the other branch at the knee. The single Channel continues down the centre of the calf muscle and passes behind the outer ankle to the outer tip of the little toe.

The Bladder Channel – functions and symptoms

The Bladder transforms waste fluids into urine, which it then excretes, helping the Kidneys to regulate water. But its Channel has a wider influence. It is an aspect of Kidney Yang, which helps in defence and supports other Organs via the associated points (see p. 117). The Kidneys "nourish the brain and spinal cord". The Bladder Channel connects with the brain and helps integrate intelligence with the functions of the nervous system.

Bladder disharmony can manifest as mental symptoms – jealousy, suspicion, obsessions, restlessness, and strained nerves.

THE BLADDER CHANNEL
Leg Greater Yang

Internal pathway symptoms (upper part): Epilepsy, nervous hyperactivity

Caution: in cases of epilepsy do not work on the head

Internal pathway symptoms (lower part): Urinary problems

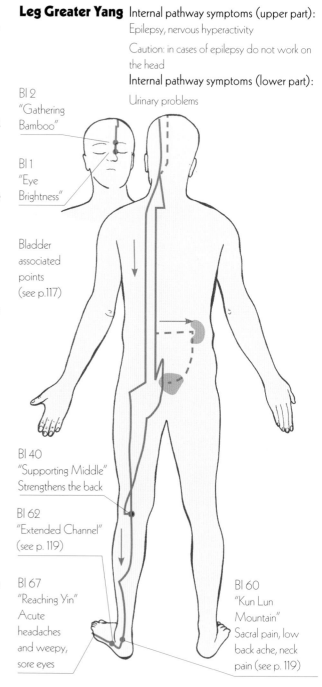

Bl 2
"Gathering Bamboo"

Bl 1
"Eye Brightness"

Bladder associated points (see p.117)

Bl 40
"Supporting Middle"
Strengthens the back

Bl 62
"Extended Channel"
(see p. 119)

Bl 67
"Reaching Yin"
Acute headaches and weepy, sore eyes

Bl 60
"Kun Lun Mountain"
Sacral pain, low back ache, neck pain (see p. 119)

The Kidney Channel pathway

This Channel begins under the little toe, near the end of the Bladder Channel, and crosses through K 1 to the inner edge of the foot. It loops behind the inside ankle bone to the heel, then rises along the inner aspect of the leg, intersecting the Spleen Channel at Sp 6, before continuing up the calf and the inner thigh. Here its pathway becomes deeper and goes to the base of the spine, where it joins the Governing Vessel. Rising internally in line with the lumbar spine it enters the Kidney, descends to the Bladder, and surfaces at the pubic area. It connects with the Directing Vessel in the lower abdomen and then rises over the body to the collarbone. Internally a branch leaves the Kidney to enter the Liver and Lung, and continues up to the throat and tongue. From the Lung another branch flows to the Heart and chest, and joins the Pericardium Channel.

The Kidneys – functions and symptoms

The Kidneys are the basis of our constitutional strength and control energy and substance in the body. They also rule the bones, open to the ear, and manifest in the head hair. Kidney Yin stores Essence, the basis of physical growth, development, and maturity. It forms "Marrow" for the brain and spinal cord, as well as bone marrow. Kidney Yang is the body's "transforming power" and supports the functions of all other Organs.

Kidney symptoms are characterized by weakness and depletion and commonly include urinary and sexual problems, aching lower back, poor memory, dizziness, hearing loss, ringing in the ears, and thinning of hair.

THE KIDNEY CHANNEL
Leg Lesser Yin

Internal pathway symptoms: Chronic sore throat, dry lungs, dry cough. Anxiety and restlessness. Backache, urinary and reproductive problems

Sp 6
"Three-Yin Meeting"

K 3
"Greater Stream"
Strengthens back,
tonifies Kidneys

K 6
"Shining Sea"
(see p. 121)

K 1
"Bubbling Spring"
(see p. 121)

CHANNEL EXERCISES
BLADDER & KIDNEYS

The role of the Bladder and Kidneys in supporting the body can lead to depletion if we push ourselves too hard. Excessive mental work can lead to brain fatigue, irritability, insomnia, and inability to relax. Excessive physical work can deplete both Ki and Essence, producing many symptoms (see p. 105). It is also important to regulate sexual activity to suit your energies, as the combination of overwork with excessive sex can provoke more serious Kidney disharmonies.

The Makko Ho exercise below rejuvenates and relaxes your body by harmonizing the kidney and bladder channels as you stretch the back and legs. Do it before sleeping. Exercise is important to balance the use of mental energy,

but rest and relaxation are equally necessary to balance physical work. In all exercises we harmonize Yin and Yang by balancing effort and relaxation.

Kidney and Bladder meridian Makko Ho stretch

Sit up as straight as possible. Stretch your legs out to the front then relax your knees and let your feet fall outward. Spread your buttocks and ease forward on to your sitting bones. If this is difficult sit on the edge of a low cushion.

Inhale and raise your arms straight above your head, palms outward. Then fold forward from your hips, keeping your chest and back extended, and exhaling as you bend. Bring your hands toward your feet, but do not try to grip your legs or pull down, Just stay in the forward bend and breathe; relax your back, neck, shoulders, arms, and legs. Remain in this position for a minute or two if you are comfortable.

Waist rotations

This simple rotation loosens the waist and stretches the back so helping the flow of Ki up and down all the Channels. It brings direct benefit to a tired, aching, sore back — a common Kidney deficiency complaint.

Stand with your feet wide apart and parallel, knees bent. Support your back behind your waist or under the back ribs. Keeping your hips and legs still, turn at the waist to face 45 degrees to one side, then fold forward over one knee and

look down. Circle smoothly across to the other knee. Lift your head and chest and face the front. Repeat the rotations for a few minutes, exhaling slowly as you bend forward and inhaling as you come up. Then change direction.

Warming the Kidneys

A natural, spontaneous way of stimulating and attracting Ki, rubbing has long been included in traditional exercise systems. Stand with your feet a shoulder-width apart, knees relaxed. Rub your hands together for a minute, holding them in front of your chest. Try to keep your shoulders relaxed. Breathe deeply. When your hands are warm, place them on your back over the Kidney area. Lean forward slightly and rub vigorously. Inhale through your mouth and blow as you exhale. Repeat once or twice. Combine this with the exercises for the Lungs (p. 82) and Triple Burner (p. 128) on cold mornings.

SHIATSU ROUTINE FOR THE BACK CHANNELS

The Heart and Small Intestine Channels on the arm, and the Bladder and Kidney Channels on the leg, represent Fire and Water, which, when in harmony, uphold and maintain constitutional strength. The Heart and Kidneys give each other mutual support. The Small Intestine and Bladder cooperate in transforming fluids and both their Channels influence the head, the neck, and the whole spine.

These four Channels flow on the inner posterior surfaces of the body and limbs and so are most easily treated with your partner lying face down.

Simplify your shiatsu

Heart and Kidney together — one meridian, "Lesser Yin"

Small Intestine

Bladder

Treat them as one meridian "Greater Yang"

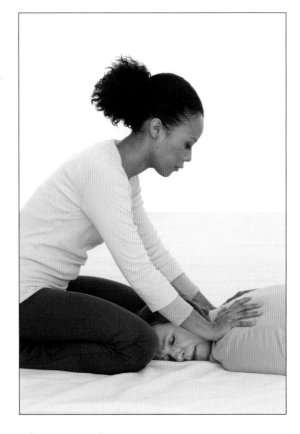

1. Preparation and positioning

Sit, knees apart, at your partner's head. Put a pillow under the chest for greater comfort, especially if your partner's neck is stiff. Relax and lean positively with your hands over the upper shoulder blade area. Allow a moment to tune in to your partner's condition.

Points for the neck and shoulder

Local points

The classical points SI 15, 14, 13, 12, and 11 (in the order of working), and SI 9 and 10 in the arm space above the armpit crease where arm and shoulder join, are locally effective points for problems of the neck and shoulder region.

2. Thumbing the Small Intestine Channel

Thumb along the SI Channel from the base of the neck to the shoulder extremity twice each side. Place your support hand on the opposite shoulder. The line runs across the top of the shoulder blade to the hollow point at the end. The Channel also runs down on to the shoulder blade (see diagram above). Work into any tsubos you find.

3. Leaning into the Small Intestine Channel

Work one side at a time, leaning with the "knife-edge" of your hand into the muscle area between the shoulder and the bone of the arm — SI 9 and 10. Use your fingers or thumbs for deeper penetration but try using the edge of the hand first: it is very effective and feels more friendly — especially important when the shoulders are stiff.

The Small Intestine Channel on the arm

As you work down the Small Intestine Channel on the arm to the fingers, the range of its influence increases. Symptoms such as headaches, sore, red eyes, acute earache, or acute gastric or urinary troubles can be eased by shiatsu along this Channel. The tsubos along the forearm to the fingers connect with other Channels, producing a calming effect on the Heart and Mind. The Bladder Channel is also affected, relaxing the spine and lower back.

4. Thumbing the Bladder Channel on the shoulders

Palm the general area between the shoulder blades, each side of the spine. Use one hand at a time or both together. Then thumb along the inner line of the Bladder Channel — the ridge of muscles about 1.5 in (4 cm) from the mid line. Work down as far as the tip of the shoulder blades, then return and give pressure along the outer line of the Channel 3 in (7.5 cm) from the mid line. Bring your weight forward as you work down.

5. Palming the Small Intestine Channel

Move to your partner's side, and remain in contact as you do so. Lift your partner's wrist, move the arm out a little and on to its edge to bring the little finger uppermost. Palm the arm from the shoulder area above the armpit down to the wrist. Relax your fingers around the arm and steady it with a gentle grip as you explore its contours.

6. "Dragon's Mouth"

This technique (see p. 44) is useful for working the SI Channel in the arm after palming. The Channel can be awkward to thumb from your position on the outside, but the bottom knuckle of your forefinger will find it naturally. Apply pressure on each tsubo.

7. Thumbing the Small Intestine Channel

Begin thumbing at SI 8 (see below and step 8 overleaf) between the elbow's bony point and the rounded tip of bone on the inner aspect of the joint. Then, move to the outer edge of the forearm (ulna) (see step 9 overleaf). After the raised prominence above the wrist, follow the Channel across the edge of the hand.

Following the Channels

Following the pathways of any arm Channel, especially the Yang Channels, can be bewildering as they can appear to deviate sharply at the elbow from one aspect to another. The Small Intestine Channel does just this. Nevertheless it is easy to reach on both upper and lower parts of the arm when your partner is lying the prone position. The 'Dragon's Mouth' technique (see step 6, p. 111) is particularly suitable on the upper arm but the thumb works best below the elbow (see below). Sit back a little to work along the outer aspect of the bone. At the wrist you will need to change position again, moving up and forward to lean down along the edge of the hand. Finish at the little finger.

8. Thumbing SI 8 at the elbow joint

9. Thumbing the Small Intestine Channel on the forearm

Small Intestine 3

The Small Intestine Channel runs between the muscle and the bone along the border between the paler and darker skin on the outer edge of the hand. SI 3 has a particularly wide influence and is situated on this line just before the knuckle of the little finger, at the tip of the crease made by folding the hand.

This point works through its own Channel, and via connections with the Bladder Channel and Governing Vessel. It strengthens the spine, relaxes muscles and tendons, calms the Mind, and helps clear judgement and decision-making. It is useful after shock or injury affecting the neck and spine, such as whiplash; also for feverish chills with shivers and spasms; for stiffness in the neck or spine, painful red eyes, ear troubles, dizziness, posterior headaches, pain in the fingers or arm, and pain or stiffness across the lower back.

SI 3 "Back Stream"

Positioning for the Heart Channel

The position for working on the Heart Channel is shown below. Place your support hand on the heart area of the back between the shoulder blades. By turning your partner's hand so the palm is facing up you will expose the inner aspect of the arm, where the Channel runs.

Treating the Heart Channel

Physical and emotional stress upset the Heart. Cold hands and feet, lethargy, spontaneous sweating, and a shiny, pale face are signs that the Heart Ki is weak. Restless, dream-disturbed sleep, hot sweaty palms, flushed cheeks, dizziness, nervousness, and irritability show that Fire and Water are unbalanced, weakening the Blood. Shiatsu for the Heart Channel can have a deeply calming effect and be beneficial to circulation.

10. Thumbing the Heart Channel

Gently grasp the upper arm near the armpit and allow your thumb to rest over the bone along the inner border of the biceps muscle. Lean with more emphasis on the thumb side and palm toward the elbow (see above). Then palm the forearm to the wrist. Repeat the technique with a more penetrating angle of the thumb.

11. Squeezing the finger

Thumb H 7 "Mind Door" found at the wrist crease (see above). This point is well known for its calming but supportive effect on the Heart and Mind. Finish by thumbing across the palm to the little finger, then gently squeeze along both sides of the finger to its tip (see above).

Rotating the limbs

Lifting and moving limbs can be hard work.
But it is easy to do if you use your body to follow
through the movement, keep your shoulders
and elbows relaxed, and take support wherever
possible – for example from your raised leg
(see below).

12. Rotating the shoulder

Pick up your partner's arm by the wrist with your nearside hand.
Scoop your outside hand under the shoulder. Lean back slightly
to stretch out the shoulder, then lift it and push it in over the
ribs, then up toward the neck. Release and stretch back to begin
again. Repeat 3 or 4 times. After the rotation try the shoulder
slash technique (see step 13, right). If the shoulders seem tight just
thumb round the inner border of the shoulder blade.

13. Slashing the shoulder blade

To "slash" the shoulder, place your partner's hand on to their back.
Ask your partner to "let go" both elbow and shoulder. Cup the
outer shoulder with one hand and place the index finger of the
other firmly alongside the shoulder blade border. Lift with the
outer hand; lean in with the other, inserting the fingers positively
under the blade for a moment. Release and repeat several times.

The Bladder Channel

Work on this Channel benefits the back, releases tension, and tonifies the Bladder and Kidneys. It also nourishes the other Organs via the "associated points" (see p. 117). Treating the lumbar and sacral areas is good for sexual and menstrual problems and can often relieve period and labour pains. Work on the leg is useful for acute back troubles and haemorrhoids, and tsubos on the foot will particularly affect the eyes, nose, neck, and head.

Distributing the body weight
Strong but safe work on the Bladder Channel, especially suitable if you are slight and the person you are working on is strong and solidly built.

14. Palming the Bladder Channel

After working on the shoulder, turn in to face your partner. Work down the Bladder Channel using your palm or the heel of your hand. Use one hand as support on the back or shoulder area and work down one side at a time. Alternatively palm both sides at once, as shown on p. 57.

15. Using your elbows

Some people with very tense or muscular backs may benefit from elbow pressure instead of thumbing. Position your elbows, relax your forearms, and gradually bring your weight forward to create perpendicular pressure. Ease back to shift your elbows, moving one a little ahead of the other as you follow the Channel down the back. You can work both sides of the spine without changing position. Relax and take your time.

16. Thumbing the sacral points

Use both thumbs together to give pressure to the sacral points. They lie in two rows, one each side of the sacrum, in line with the main inner pathway of the Bladder Channel, and the other even closer to the mid line (see p. 104). Shiatsu on the sacrum can help lower back pain, menstrual pain, and problems of the bladder and sexual organs.

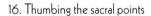

The Bladder "associated points"

Twelve classically established points along the Bladder Channel relate directly to the twelve inner Organs. They are found along the inner line of the Bladder Channel down the back in three regions that correspond to the regions of the Triple Burner (see p. 125). In the upper region, between the shoulder blades, level with the bony process of the 3rd, 4th, and 5th thoracic vertebrae, are points for the Lungs, Pericardium, and Heart. These are the Organs of the chest influencing circulation of Ki and Blood. The next two points also help circulation, especially Bl 17 (the Diaphragm "associated point"), a dynamic, strengthening, and regulating point for Blood.

In the middle region, level with the 9th to 12th thoracic vertebrae, are four associated points – for the Liver, Gall Bladder, Spleen, and Stomach. These work on the digestion, absorption, and distribution of nutrients. The lower region is concerned with storage of reserves, sexual functions, drainage, and elimination. It is dominated by the Kidneys, with points level with the 2nd lumbar vertebra at the narrowest part of the waist, just above the hips. Just above are the points for the Triple Burner; these help regulate fluids. Those of the Large Intestine, Small Intestine, Bladder, anus, and sacral region are found further down.

All these points carry Ki directly to the Organs, so they are sometimes called "Transporting Points". They can also be used for diagnosis. If an Organ is out of balance its associated point can become tender or sensitive to pressure. These points will help you develop an insight into your partner's general condition and so give effective treatments.

THE ASSOCIATED POINTS

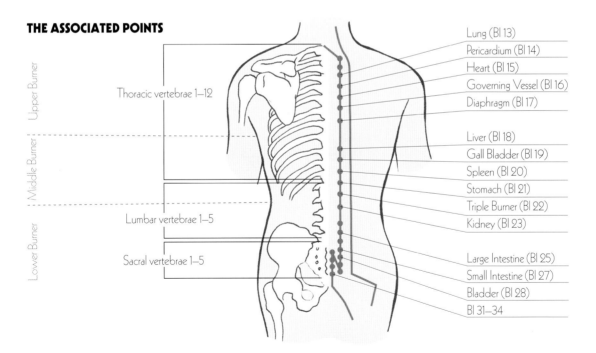

Upper Burner

Middle Burner

Lower Burner

Thoracic vertebrae 1–12

Lumbar vertebrae 1–5

Sacral vertebrae 1–5

Lung (Bl 13)
Pericardium (Bl 14)
Heart (Bl 15)
Governing Vessel (Bl 16)
Diaphragm (Bl 17)

Liver (Bl 18)
Gall Bladder (Bl 19)
Spleen (Bl 20)
Stomach (Bl 21)
Triple Burner (Bl 22)
Kidney (Bl 23)

Large Intestine (Bl 25)
Small Intestine (Bl 27)
Bladder (Bl 28)
Bl 31–34

Work on the legs

To finish this routine, work down the Bladder and Kidney Channels on each leg. You can do this most effectively by treating first the Bladder Channel on the nearside and then, from the same position, leaning over to work down the Kidney Channel on the inner aspect of the opposite leg. Keep your support hand in touch with the sacral or lower lumbar region. Remember to change sides and work both Channels on both legs.

Preparation

Check that your partner's ankles are relaxed so the feet contact the floor when you lean on their legs. If not, provide support with a small cushion or rolled towel.

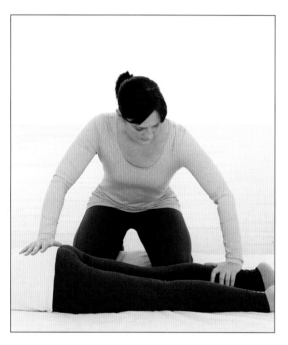

17. Palming the Bladder Channel

Lean with the palm or heel of the hand over the mid line of the thigh. Begin under the buttocks (see p. 60) and work toward the knee, calf, and ankle. Keep a wide base and avoid over-reaching.

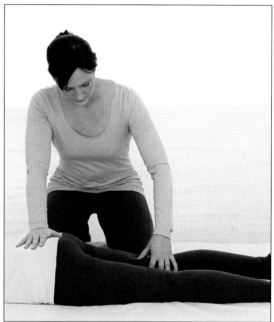

18. Thumbing the Bladder Channel

Thumb the Channel from the same position. Half way down the calf the Bladder Channel deviates outward slightly to run in the groove between the Achilles tendon and the ankle and on to the outside of the foot (see step 19, facing page). You can thumb the Channel right along the edge of the foot to the little toe or you may prefer to stop at the ankle and treat the feet separately after working the Kidney Channel (see p. 121).

The Bladder Channel on the foot

The last section of the Bladder Channel influences the distant parts where the Channel begins.

Bl 60 ("Kun Lun Mountain") in the hollow between the ankle and the Achilles tendon strengthens the whole spine from sacrum to neck and helps ease a stiff neck and posterior headaches. It also helps to relieve menstrual pain, labour pains, and burning urination.

Bl 62 ("Extended Channel"), 1 in (2.5 cm) below the ankle tip, brings benefits to the whole back and relaxes the leg muscles. It also calms the mind and clears the eyes, helping reduce restlessness and insomnia if stimulated strongly (see also K 6, p. 121).

The Bladder Channel in the leg

The Bladder Channel in the foot

19. Thumbing the Bladder Channel on the foot

Work the Bladder points on the foot (see left) and explore for other tsubos, supporting the ankle with one hand, while working along the Channel with the extended thumb of the other (see above). Don't get so involved with detail that you forget to relax and lean from your Hara. Finish by squeezing and pulling the little toe.

The remaining points, in the hollows between the muscle and bones along the edge of the foot, relieve congestion in the head, relax the neck, and calm the mind. They also clear the eyes when they are inflamed or blurry from the effect of wind, pollen, or acute infection.

Treating the Kidneys

In addition to the common symptoms of Kidney deficiency (see p. 105) further symptom patterns characterize a weakness of either Yin or Yang Kidney functions.

Kidney Yang weakness manifests in fatigue, weak legs, cold feelings, frequent profuse urination or incontinence, low libido, or in men, a tendency to impotence.

Weak Kidney Yin produces dryness and thirst, night sweats, insomnia, chronic sore throats, flushed cheeks, scanty menstruation in women, and premature ejaculation in men.

It is important to treat the Bladder Channel in all Kidney problems, especially weakness of Yang. Kidney Yin deficiencies respond well to work on the leg, especially the Kidney points near the ankle. Rest and special exercises, such as Tai Chi, Chi Kung, or yoga are traditionally recommended for Kidney depletion.

20. Palming the Kidney Channel

After palming and thumbing the Bladder Channel on the near leg, lean across to the opposite leg, to work on the Kidney Channel. Keep your support hand on the sacrum and palm down the inner aspect of the back of the thigh and leg.

21. Thumbing the Kidney Channel

To tonify the Channel, relax, and work down slowly with the thumb. Feel for the deepest or most open tsubos and take time to let your pressure penetrate. Hold each one for several breaths. K 3 is the last point on the leg, behind the inner ankle (see above). Repeat your work on the leg Channels on the other side. Then move on to the Bladder Channel (p. 119) and the Kidney Channel (facing page) on the foot.

Treating Kidney Yin deficiency

When in harmony, Yang is above and should go downward, Yin is below and moves upward, as in the normal direction of the Channels. Deficiency of Yin often causes the Yang Ki of the body to rise or rebel upward, causing unpleasant dry or hot symptoms in the head and disturbing the mind.

Typical patterns of Kidney Yin deficiency include chronic sore throat, thirst, flushed cheeks, and dry, sore eyes, restlessness, and insomnia. All the Kidney points around the inner ankle and on the foot tend to strengthen Yin and rectify this imbalance.

Kidney 1

This is another point that calms Yang and tonifies or strengthens the Yin. It is useful for someone in a particularly manic or disturbed state of restlessness, but it can also be helpful in shock or fainting, with headaches or nosebleeds, or exhaustion from heat.

K 1 is in the middle of the front part of the sole at the convergence of the lines made when the foot is flexed. Thumb systematically over the whole of the sole for a strengthening and calming influence (see also pp. 171).

Kidney 1

Ki 1

Kidney 6

Located in the hollow about 1 in (2.5 cm) below the tip of the inner ankle, this point sends Yin influence upward. It moistens the throat and eyes, calms the mind, and promotes sleep. If the person is particularly restless and tense, work more strongly first on the Bladder Channels, particularly Bl 62 (see p. 119).

Kidney 6 "Shining Sea"

22. Using the knuckles

This is a pleasant and effective alternative method if your thumbs are tired, or just for a change. Clasp under your partner's ankle with one hand as shown above, keeping your hand on the floor for support. Then knead the whole underside of your partner's foot with the folded finger knuckles of the other hand, using your weight to apply a firm pressure.

8. THE SIDE CHANNELS

PERICARDIUM (HEART PROTECTOR), TRIPLE BURNER, GALL BLADDER, LIVER

The Channels of these four Organs form the last part of the cycle of Ki (see p. 74), flowing on the sides of the body between all the other Channels. The Pericardium and Triple Burner assist and protect. The Pericardium works for the Heart. Reflecting its classical name, it is the "Heart's Protector". It mediates in social interaction, "like a minister to the monarch" preventing harm from emotional excesses as well as from extreme environmental heat and fevers. The Triple Burner meridian helps to protect the body by regulating surface defences. As an organ it has no precise form, but harmonizes the functions of the body's upper, middle, and lower regions (see pp. 126–27). Its Ki assists transformation and regulates fluids in each region, co-operating with the Lungs, Spleen, and Kidneys. It acts as an avenue for Kidney Ki to replenish the other Channels, warming and protecting the body surface.

The Pericardium and the Triple Burner both belong to the Fire element. Their "Minister" Fire is associated with Kidney Yang, the "Life-Gate Fire" of Mei Mon, and the Hara.

The Liver and Gall Bladder belong to the Wood element. Materially they store and distribute pure substances. The Liver stores Blood, releasing it to the muscles for activity. The Gall Bladder stores bile, which it releases for digestion.

Organs of creative action, skillful planning, wise judgement, and appropriate decisions, the Liver and Gall Bladder encompass destiny. Courageous decisions are the gift of the Gall Bladder. The Liver enables Ki to flow freely so that all body functions are smooth, and by its influence on planning, foresight and adaptability, makes an easy path through life. The Gall Bladder Channel influences all the bi-lateral joints, helping physical mobility.

The pathways for these four Channels are illustrated on pp. 125 and 130–31; the Channel exercises are on pp. 128–29 and 132–33. The routine begins on p. 134.

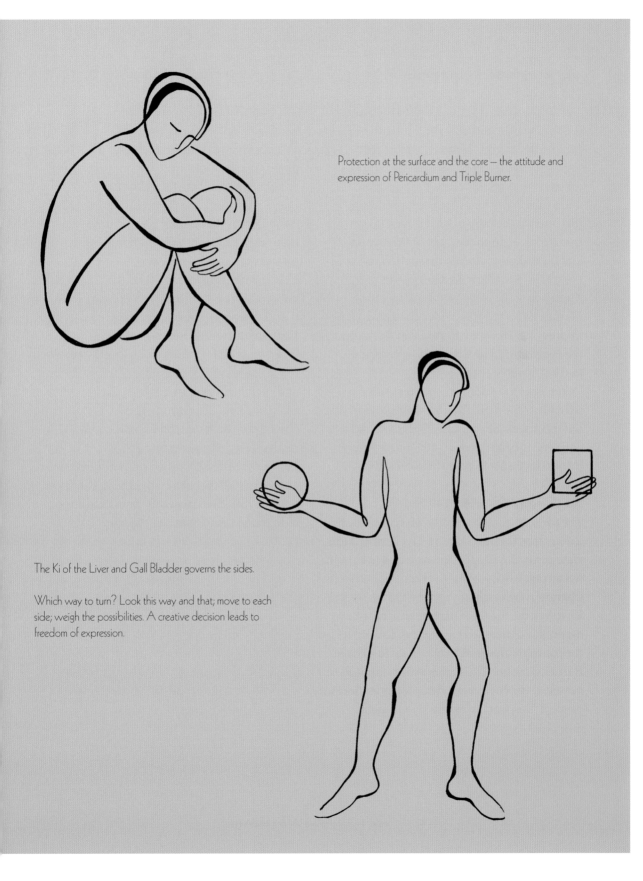

Protection at the surface and the core — the attitude and expression of Pericardium and Triple Burner.

The Ki of the Liver and Gall Bladder governs the sides.

Which way to turn? Look this way and that; move to each side; weigh the possibilities. A creative decision leads to freedom of expression.

The Pericardium Channel pathway

This Channel begins in the middle of the chest at the Pericardium. A branch descends internally through the diaphragm to the Upper, Middle, and Lower "Burners" – the three regions of the Triple Burner (see p. 127).

From the starting point a branch of the main Channel crosses the chest to emerge just outside the nipple. It then ascends on the surface around the front of the armpit and flows down the arm, through the biceps muscle. At the elbow crease it passes just to the inside of the biceps tendon (the Lung Channel is on the other side), then down the middle of the front of the forearm, between the Heart and Lung Channels (see pp. 100 and 80), to the wrist.

It crosses the middle of the palm to P 8 where it divides. The main Channel continues to the outer corner of the middle fingernail, and a connecting branch goes to the fourth finger to join the Triple Burner Channel at TB 1.

The changing view of the Pericardium

The early classics constantly referred to the five Yin and the six Yang Organs. The Pericardium was seen as the Heart's protector and assistant, not an organ in its own right. Some points on its Channel were originally ascribed to the Heart. However, the theory of the twelve Channels eventually demanded a symmetry that led to the pairing of the Pericardium with the Triple Burner Channel. Their relationship is not close, however, and their categorization under the Fire element (see p. 21) is for different reasons.

The Pericardium Channel – functions and symptoms

The Pericardium is described as the Heart's "ambassador", bringing joy and happiness, helping to communicate our feelings, and protecting the Heart from emotional pain when relationships become stressful. To achieve this, the Pericardium Channel calms the Mind and balances the emotions, especially when there are relationship problems and break-ups (heartaches and heartbreaks).

As the Heart belongs to the Fire element it is vulnerable to extra Heat. The Pericardium's role as "Heart Protector" extends to absorbing Heat, to protect the Heart from attacks of fever. Most of the points along this Channel reduce hot symptoms associated with Heart or Blood disorders, and its last three points are specifically used for high fevers with great thirst, delirium, hallucinations, and restlessness, or prostration (e.g. sunstroke). The Pericardium Channel has a wide influence on the chest. It eases chest tightness, stuffiness, or pains, whether caused by emotional stress, indigestion (heartburn), or phlegm.

THE PERICARDIUM (HEART PROTECTOR) CHANNEL
Arm Terminal Yin

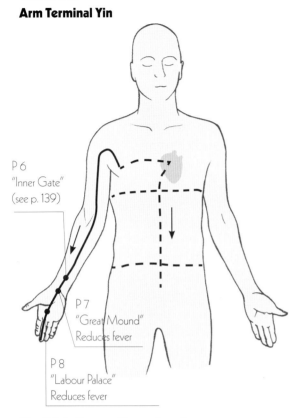

P 6
"Inner Gate"
(see p. 139)

P 7
"Great Mound"
Reduces fever

P 8
"Labour Palace"
Reduces fever

THE TRIPLE BURNER CHANNEL
Arm Lesser Yang

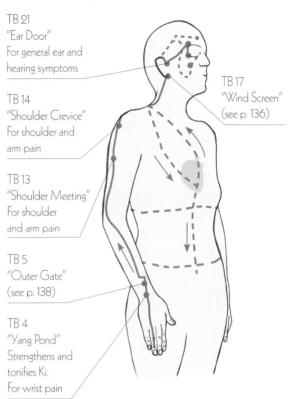

TB 21
"Ear Door"
For general ear and
hearing symptoms

TB 17
"Wind Screen"
(see p. 136)

TB 14
"Shoulder Crevice"
For shoulder and
arm pain

TB 13
"Shoulder Meeting"
For shoulder
and arm pain

TB 5
"Outer Gate"
(see p. 138)

TB 4
"Yang Pond"
Strengthens and
tonifies Ki.
For wrist pain

The Triple Burner Channel pathway

Beginning on the fourth finger, by the outside corner of the nail, the Triple Burner Channel passes between the knuckles of the fourth and fifth fingers to the wrist. From here it ascends between the two bones of the forearm (radius and ulna), through the tip of the elbow, and up the back of the arm to the shoulder. Behind the top of the shoulder it joins the Small Intestine and the Governing Vessel Channels. Then it rises over the shoulder to the collarbone region, descends internally to the Pericardium in the Upper Burner, and then to the abdomen and the Middle and Lower Burners (see p. 127). Re-emerging from the chest at the collarbone, the Triple Burner Channel ascends the side of the neck and round the back of the ear. One branch rises internally to meet the Gall Bladder Channel on the forehead, then descends to join the Small Intestine Channel on the cheek. The superficial branch continues to the front of the ear and crosses to the outer corner of the eyebrow, where it joins the Gall Bladder Channel again, next in the cycle of energy flow (see p. 74).

The Triple Burner Channel – functions and symptoms

Symptoms of the Yang Channels often relate to their superficial pathways, and are connected with their role in defending the body from acute disease and environmental influences. The Triple Burner is no exception. Symptoms of this Channel include sore, red eyes, acute ear troubles or pain behind the ear, sore or swollen throat, and pains in the shoulder or arm, also symptoms of chills and fevers, either acute or chronically recurring, sometimes with spontaneous sweating.

The Triple Burner transforms and regulates body fluids. It also assists the Kidneys, so treating it can move the Ki in the body's interior, especially the lower region. It can help when there is abdominal swelling and discomfort, sometimes with urination difficulties or constipation.

It also helps in weakness that is combined with an inability to stabilize body temperature and a susceptibility to infections and fevers. However, it is usually more effective to treat imbalances of the Three Burners by treating the Channels of the relevant Organs in each particular region.

The Triple Burner controversy

The Triple Burner has been the subject of much discussion and controversy in Chinese medicine. Some early classics described it as an Organ like other Yang Organs, with particular involvement in absorbing, metabolizing, and excreting fluids, but with no specific location (see diagram opposite, left hand column). Others maintained that it was a generalization of the structure and energies of the upper, middle, and lower parts of the body – the "three regions" or "burners" – which included the functions of the Organs within each region (see opposite, right hand column).

Yet another classic (see quote on the facing page) described it as an Organ with "a name but no form" and developed a more integrated view of the Triple Burner as an "avenue of Ki", assisting in all transformations by conducting basic, constitutional Ki from Mei Mon, the "Life-Gate" in the Hara (see p. 51), to the other Organs. It helps extract Ki from air and food and supports the Lungs, Spleen, and Kidneys in the Upper, Middle, and Lower Burners respectively. Similarly, the Triple Burner conveys stored constitutional Ki to the twelve Channels when they are depleted, supplying energy for the body's defence in times of illness or stress. In this model the Lower Burner includes the "storing up" of constitutional Ki as Essence by the Kidneys.

The role of the Liver

Some interpretations of the "bodily regions" model of the Triple Burner describe the Liver as part of the Lower Burner because of its strong influence on moving Ki and Blood in this area. The Liver has as much effect on the reproductive organs as do the Kidneys. Physically, however, it is in the middle region.

Understanding the Triple Burner

Consider the Triple Burner as a framework for understanding human physiology in the traditional Chinese way. Remember to think of both the general and the specific roles of all

THE "FLUID-REGULATING" MODEL OF THE TRIPLE BURNER

The Upper Burner is compared to a mist, as the Lungs disperse fluids to moisten the whole body, especially the skin.

The Middle Burner is compared to a muddy pool or swamp, steaming and bubbling like the activity of the Stomach and Spleen in digesting and separating food and fluids.

The Lower Burner is described as a drainage ditch, separating clean from dirty fluids and carrying away the waste (SI, BI and K functions)

THE "THREE BODILY REGIONS" MODEL OF THE TRIPLE BURNER

The upper region includes the chest, neck, and head, and the functions of the Lungs, Heart, and Pericardium. It "receives but does not expel".

The middle region comprises the area between the diaphragm and the navel and includes the functions of the Liver, Gall Bladder, Stomach, and Spleen. It "moves and transforms".

The lower region starts below the navel and includes the functions of the Large and Small Intestines, Bladder, and Kidneys. This region "excretes but does not receive".

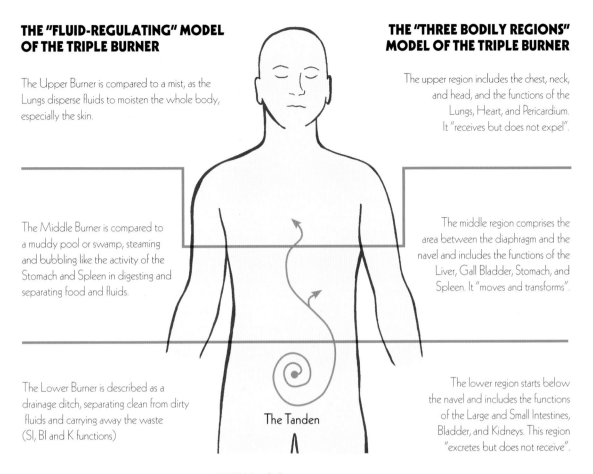

The Tanden

"Avenue of Ki" Model

The Classic of Difficulties describes the Hara centre, or Tanden as the front focus of the "moving Ki between the Kidneys". According to the "avenue of Ki" model of the Triple Burner, this activates transformations in the three "burners" and nourishes all the Organs and their Channels, as shown symbolically by the arrow in the illustration above.

the Organs, and to see their overlapping and interacting functions as part of a harmonious system. Understanding this synthesis can help you interpret symptoms and therefore treat people more effectively.

> *"The Triple Burner is the avenue of food and drink, the beginning and the end of Ki."*
> CLASSIC OF DIFFICULTIES (C.100 AD)

CHANNEL EXERCISES
PERICARDIUM & TRIPLE BURNER

The first exercise on this page is a Makko Ho stretch to stretch and stimulate the Pericardium and Triple Burner Channels. Adapted from the posture of protection (see below right), it symbolizes emotional defensiveness, dejection, or shyness, and signifies huddling for warmth and protection from the elements.

The exercises that follow enhance our positive capacity to generate warmth and protection by building Ki through breathing,

relaxed movement, and mental focus. The last in the sequence encourages an easy, rhythmic movement that loosens obstructed Ki, and lifts the spirit. The Pericardium influences circulation of Ki in the chest, the Triple Burner in the ribs and lower abdomen, and the Gall Bladder along the sides of the body and in the joints generally. These all assist the Liver, which governs the smooth flow of Ki throughout the body.

Makko Ho stretch for Pericardium (Heart Protector) and Triple Burner Channels

Sit up straight, cross-legged. Tuck your inside foot in close to the groin. Cross your arms and hold around your knees. Exhale, and bend forward from the hips (see above). Tuck in your elbows and relax your upper body, head, and neck. Keep your buttocks on the floor and your pelvis relaxed. Breathe into the Hara. Exhale as you sit up, cross your arms and legs the other way, and repeat.

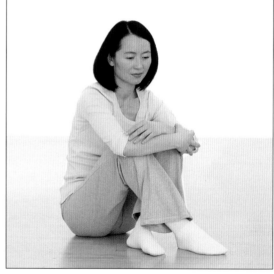

Posture of Protection

The Makko Ho stretch (see left) develops from the expression of the Pericardium and Triple Burner Channels (see above).

Rubbing hands

Pericardium 8, "Labour Palace", in the middle of the palms is regarded as an important focus for Ki. Rub your hands together in a relaxed but intent and purposeful way, keeping your breathing easy and deep. This soon produces warmth in the hands, increases their healing potential, and encourages Ki to circulate through your whole body.

Stimulating the Channels by beating

Form a loosely clenched fist and, keeping your wrist relaxed, beat your chest firmly from the centre of your breastbone (sternum) up and across to the front of your shoulder, then down the Pericardium Channel on the front of your arm to your palm. Turn your arm to beat its outer surface – the Triple Burner Channel – from wrist up to the shoulders. Finish by lifting your arm and beating down the Gall Bladder Channel on the side of the ribs.

Arm swinging

Stand with your feet wide apart and parallel. Sink down a little, then relax your pelvis, and tuck your tailbone in. Turn your knees out slightly. Now turn from the waist first to one side then the other. Let your arms swing naturally. Increase the movement, and eventually your arms will swing right round and slap your waist on the opposite sides.

The Gall Bladder Channel

This Channel begins just outside the outer corner of the eye, loops down and up to the forehead just within the hairline, and descends behind the ear to the corner of the skull. It then returns to the forehead above the centre of the eye and contours the head to the bottom of the skull at GB 20. It continues down the neck behind the shoulder to connect with the Governing Vessel at GV 14, then crosses over the shoulder. The Channel descends the side of the body along the rib margin to the waist and pelvic crest before going deeper to meet the Bladder Channel at the sacrum. At GB 30 it re-emerges and continues down the outside of the leg, in front of the ankle, ending on the outside of the fourth toe. Internal branches connect with the Stomach Channel (on the jaw) and the Small Intestine Channel, and join the Liver and Gall Bladder Organs.

Gall Bladder Channel – functions and symptoms

The Gall Bladder stores and secretes bile, which aids digestion, especially of fats. People with poor Gall Bladder function have difficulty digesting rich, fatty foods. This coincides with the Western medical view. Stagnation of Ki or Heat in the Gall Bladder can produce pain under the ribs, nausea and vomiting, a bitter or sour taste in the mouth, and yellow colour in the eyes.

The Gall Bladder influences the sides of the body and blockages or imbalances of the Gall Bladder Channel manifest in temple headaches, eye and ear pain, stiffness or pain in the jaw, shoulders, ribs, hips, or knee and ankle joints.

THE GALL BLADDER CHANNEL
Leg Lesser Yang

GB 21
"Shoulder Well"
(see p. 137)

Caution: Avoid strong shiatsu on top of shoulders in early pregnancy

GB 30
"Jumping Circle"
For hip pain and sciatica

GB 34
"Yang Mound Spring"
Relaxes muscles and tendons.
For all stiffness and spasms (see p. 141)

GB 40
"Ruined Mound"
(see p. 141)

GB 12
"Final Bone"
For acute side headaches, disturbed sleep (see p. 168)

GB 20
"Wind Pool"
Major point for many head symptoms (see p. 136)

THE LIVER CHANNEL
Leg Terminal Yin

Internal pathway symptoms (upper parts)

Headaches at the top of the head, dizziness and disturbed vision, sensation of obstruction in the throat, asthma, stiffness and oppression (in the chest), pre-menstrual syndrome

Internal pathway symptoms (lower parts)

For irregular or painful periods; bloated abdomen, irritation, pain or swelling in the genitals

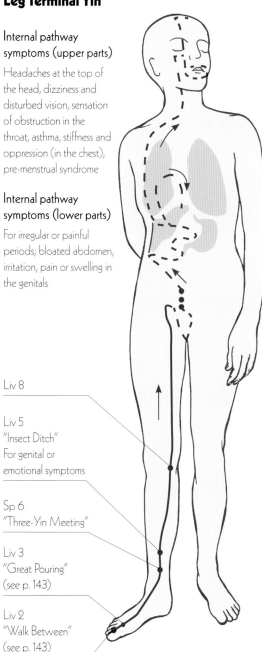

Liv 8

Liv 5
"Insect Ditch"
For genital or emotional symptoms

Sp 6
"Three-Yin Meeting"

Liv 3
"Great Pouring"
(see p. 143)

Liv 2
"Walk Between"
(see p. 143)

The Liver Channel pathway

Beginning by the inside of the big toenail the Liver Channel crosses the top of the foot, passes in front of the inside ankle and up the inner aspect of the leg through Sp 6 close behind the edge of the bone. It continues past the knee along the inner thigh to the groin and pubic region, where it circulates the external genitals. It connects with the Directing Vessel in the lower abdomen and continues up around the Stomach to enter both the Liver and Gall Bladder. Connecting with two surface points on the ribs, the Channel then dips into the ribcage, runs up through the throat, opening to the eye, and ends at the crown of the head where it connects with the Governing Vessel. A branch circles the mouth.

From within the liver, another internal branch reaches the Lungs, and this restarts the cycle of Ki (see p. 74).

The functions of the Liver

The two principal functions of the Liver are storing Blood and helping all body functions run smoothly by spreading the Ki. The Liver also controls tendons and ligaments, and releases Blood to nourish these during activity, so that the joints and muscles work smoothly. Liver Blood also nourishes the eyes, to which the Liver "opens". The Blood returns to the Liver during rest.

Blockage of Ki causes Liver-related problems – aches, pains, and irregularity – in many parts of the body. The wide-ranging influence of Liver Ki can be seen by studying the course of its Channel.

CHANNEL EXERCISES
GALL BLADDER & LIVER

The Liver guides our destiny; its role is associated with organization and planning. Its influence on the eyes not only relates to good sight but symbolically to insight and foresight. In this it is assisted by the Gall Bladder, with its influence over good judgement and decision making. The Liver has the overview while the Gall Bladder looks after the details.

Frustrations and difficulties can lead to anger, the powerful Liver emotion. Expressed appropriately, this can overcome obstacles and lead to creative solutions. However, unresolved difficulties block Liver Ki, and this results in depressions. Irritability and unwarranted aggression come when the naturally expansive Wood energies find no proper outlet and rebel upward, often producing physical symptoms such as headaches. Cowardice, timidity, and becoming "bogged-down" in details indicate weakness of the Gall Bladder.

Makko Ho stretch for Liver and Gall Bladder Channels

Sit up with your legs stretched wide. Turn at the waist to face your left foot. Brace your left hand on the floor behind to lift your trunk and spine. Now wrap your right arm around your chest and ribs and inhale as you raise your left arm. Exhale slowly and lower your trunk and left arm in line with your right leg. Rest your arm over your head and relax for 2 or 3 breaths. Come out of the position and repeat on the other side.

Gentle swing turn

Relaxed stretches and exercises in easy coordinated movement benefit the Liver and Gall Bladder generally. Gentle "swing turns" (see above) open the sides and move the Ki. The exercises on these pages echo the symbolic gesture on p.123 – "weighing up the alternatives, considering the options".

Easy arm swings

Stand straight in a relaxed posture, with your knees and hips loose. Gaze toward the horizon. Now begin a gentle bouncing movement from the knee and ankle joints, dipping and rising in a rhythm equivalent to your relaxed walking pace. Let your arms swing according to the same rhythm, driven by your body movement. Your feet stay planted, and your arms swing gently with each bounce, never above chest height. Make it easy, as if you could "walk" all day, enjoying the movement, never needing to arrive, already there.

Try the same exercise, but swinging your arms together. Feel your arms falling under the influence of gravity after each upswing, with only the little bounce helping the movement continue, like a pendulum motion. Breathe naturally. Continue the exercise for several minutes.

Twisting arcs

This exercise in flowing movement and coordination gently opens the sides of the body and moves the waist. Take a wider stance than in the previous exercises, with your hands held in front, palms upward at the level of your groin. Imagine that a ball is balanced on each hand and carry one ball out behind you, past the hip. Take it in a whole arc round, up, and to the front, over your head, back, and round again to the starting position. Keep your palm up and breathe normally. Repeat on the other side.

SHIATSU ROUTINE FOR THE SIDE CHANNELS

The side position is especially useful for elderly people, pregnant women, and people with certain kinds of back pain, breathing troubles, or indigestion. It is particularly good for treating the four Channels in this chapter.

The Triple Burner and Gall Bladder have a strong influence on the sides of the body. They are implicated in many one-sided complaints or injuries. The Pericardium and Liver Channels share an involvement in emotional expression. For sensitive people the giver's position behind the receiver can feel supportive and non-confrontational, while permitting some deeply effective shiatsu.

Simplify theory and practice

Triple Burner and Gall Bladder together, "Lesser Yang", one meridian path

Pericardium (Heart Protector) and Liver; two channels, sometimes only one, "Terminal Yin"

1. Supporting the shoulder

Use a pillow to support your partner's head. Find the most stable position for your partner by bringing the lower shoulder forward slightly to rest on the ground, and folding the top leg forward in front of the outstretched lower leg.

Kneel close by your partner's back, resting your nearside hand on the shoulder and placing your other between the shoulder blades, the area corresponding with the Heart and Pericardium. Pause for a moment.

2. Rotating the shoulder

Insert your arm under your partner's armpit to support the front of the shoulder. Clasp the shoulder with both hands and begin to move it slowly in circles. Use your Hara and your body movement to follow and feel the limits of the motion and rotate the joint more widely — a few times in each direction.

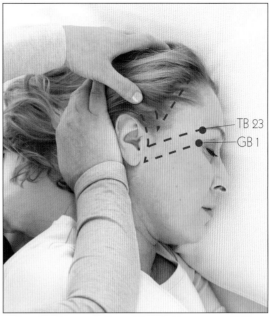

TB 23
GB 1

4. Thumbing the Triple Burner and Gall Bladder Channels

Begin at TB 23, the small hollow near the outer end of the eyebrow, and follow the path of the Triple Burner (see p. 125) down to the front of the ear then around to TB 17. Return to GB 1, level with the outer corner of the eye, and thumb this Channel down to the hollow in front of the ear, then up to the forehead and back around the ear. Work a little outside the TB Channel as shown, to GB 12 at the corner of the skull.

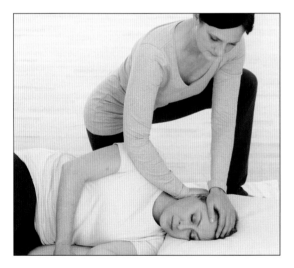

3. Palming the side of the head

Palming the side of the head opens both of the Yang Channels (Triple Burner and Gall Bladder) that cross it. Kneel up and step forward with your outer leg. Support your partner with the thigh of your other leg. Place your palms comfortably on your partner's head. Lean and palm gently around the side of the head.

Positioning the support hand

In this part of the routine your nearside hand always plays the supporting role. Tuck your elbow against your partner's shoulder and place your support hand behind the head while your active hand works on parts in front of the ear.

Shiatsu on the head

Even on the head there are subtle hollows and dents that correspond to the joints in the skull. Feel with sensitivity for these points as you go. Use relaxed leaning pressure into those you can feel. The skin and underlying membranes and muscles of the head are very lively and responsive. This makes work on the head very rewarding.

TB 17 ("Wind Screen")

Located in the hollow between the corners of the jawbone and skull, behind the ear lobe, this sensitive but important point is useful for all ear troubles including pain from exposure to wind – hence its name. Press gently but firmly with the tip of your thumb or forefinger.

GB 20 ("Wind Pool")

Located under the skull in the large hollow between the muscles, this is one of the most important points for the head. With a strong clearing and dispersing action, GB 20 is helpful for all headaches, including migraine. Use it also for eye troubles, ear problems, or stuffiness, pain, or blockage of the nose and sinuses, acute or chronic.

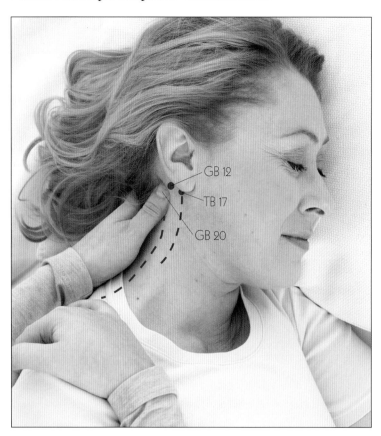

GB 12

TB 17

GB 20

5. Working the neck

Sit back slightly and cup your support hand around the shoulder, then lean back a little to "open" the neck. With the fingers of your working hand you can give quite firm pressure to the tsubos under the base of the skull, particularly GB 12 and GB 20 (see left). Work down the neck, at first just resting your thumb across the sterno-cleido-mastoid muscle using the relaxed weight of your arm. Then, working a little more firmly with extended thumb, give pressure behind the muscle to the TB Channel (see p. 125). Return to the base of the skull and follow the GB Channel (see p. 130), leaning with the thumb in a similar way into the groove between the neck muscles.

6. Thumbing Triple Burner and Gall Bladder Channels on top of the shoulder

Squat and turn to face your partner's feet. Rest your near hand over the head, curling your fingers under the base of the skull. With the thumb of the other hand work the TB and GB Channels across the top of the shoulder, inching along from the corner of the neck as far as the bony extremity.

Caution: GB 21, which is at the top of the shoulder, near the neck, should not be pressed during the early stages of pregnancy or whenever there is threatened miscarriage. It is useful, however, during labour as part of an "inducing" treatment.

7. Loosening the shoulder blade

Kneeling alongside your partner's back, place your hands around the shoulder. Rock the joint loosely between your hands and feel for the inner border of the shoulder blade so that you can curl and insert your fingers a little way underneath. Hook your fingers firmly under the shoulder blade, and supporting the front with equal pressure, lift up, out, and away from the spine by leaning back and opening your own body — a lovely releasing sensation for the receiver, which you can repeat a couple of times.

Treating the Triple Burner Channel

To treat this Channel, rest the arm along your partner's side, wrist over the hip. Kneel up behind, with your knees wide spaced, and steady your partner's shoulder with your supporting hand. The Channel runs just to the rear of the mid line of the shoulder muscle (deltoid), down to the bony point of the elbow.

TB 5 ("Outer Gate")

The most versatile, wide acting point of the Triple Burner Channel is found 2 in (5 cm) above the wrist, between the bones (see below left). Useful in acute, feverish conditions, with chills, sore throat, and sweating, and as a "distant point" for earache, side headaches, swollen glands, and stiff neck, TB 5 is also good for pain in the ribs, shoulder, or wrist.

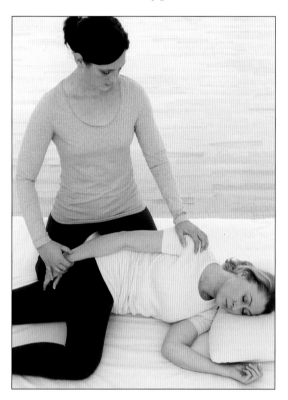

8. Thumbing the Triple Burner Channel on the arm

Palm the outer arm from the shoulder muscle to the wrist. Then kneel back slightly to thumb the Channel in the upper arm. To follow the Channel from the elbow, kneel up close and lean directly down, thumbing along the space between the two bones of the forearm as shown here (TB 5), continuing to the hollow at the wrist where the tendons of the hand converge.

9. Finishing the Triple Burner Channel

Continue toward the space between the knuckles of the 4th and 5th fingers and finish by squeezing the sides of the 4th finger.

The Pericardium Channel

This Channel runs right through the mid line of the biceps muscle on the upper arm, passing to the inside of the tendon at the elbow. Then it runs along the middle inside aspect of the forearm, between the two prominent tendons above the wrist (P 6), across the middle of the palm, and along the middle finger.

Start work on this Channel by rotating the shoulder (see p. 135), finishing with your partner's arm across your lap.

Pericardium 6 ("Inner Gate")

This point is situated approximately 2 in (5 cm) above the inner wrist crease, between the two prominent tendons of the lower arm.

It has a strong influence on the whole chest area, and "harmonizes the Stomach". Use this point when indigestion causes nausea, acidity, and heartburn. It is also valuable as first aid for morning sickness and travel sickness.

P 6 moves Ki and Blood and calms the Mind. It helps anxiety, depression, and all kinds of emotional problems, especially when accompanied by tightness, heaviness, or pain in the chest. It also relieves pre-menstrual syndrome with distention or pain in the breasts.

P 6

10. Palming the Channel

At first palm the Channel with your thumb laid flat across the inner arm, exerting general pressure while your fingers support behind. Return to the top and thumb the Channel at a more penetrating angle. Keep your shoulder relaxed.

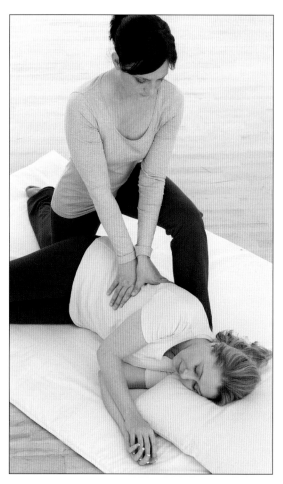

Positioning for the Gall Bladder Channel

While working down this Channel in the leg, your supporting hand can rest usefully on the classical point GB 30 situated on the outside of the buttock, just above and behind the prominent hip bone. It acts on all the leg joints and also benefits the lower back. It has a strengthening and comforting effect. Sciatic pain often follows the path of the Gall Bladder Channel. In this case, palming is the best general technique – use your thumbs sparingly if the pain is bad.

11. "Dragon's Mouth" technique for the ribs

This two-handed version of the "Dragon's Mouth" (see p. 44) is ideal for working the GB Channel on the sides and helps move Ki in the chest. After working down the arm, lift and rotate it once or twice more then place it down comfortably in front. Kneel up and lean with both hands spread over the side of the ribs (see above), as you work down from the armpit to the waist. Keep both hands together and give your partner time to breathe with the movement. Be firm yet relaxed — light pressure is ticklish.

Positioning for working the GB Channel

Step across your partner's legs as shown. Palm down the centre of the outer aspect of the limb from the hip to the ankle joint.

GB 34 ("Yang Mound Spring")

On the outside of the leg, 2 in (5 cm) below the kneecap, GB 34 is found in the hollow immediately below and just in front of the head of the fibula, a small bony prominence – the "Yang Mound" of the point's name.

This point helps the Liver smooth the flow of Ki. It is generally relaxing and has a special action on all tendons and muscles. It helps in sprains and strains, pain and stiffness of any joints, muscular spasms, abdominal cramps, and constipation. It also benefits Gall Bladder symptoms such as biliousness and indigestion pains below the ribs.

GB 40 ("Ruined Mound")

Immediately below and to the front of the outer ankle bone, GB 40 strengthens the Gall Bladder and is useful for many problems occurring along the Channel. It is a good "distant point" for knee and hip pains, rib pains, stiff neck, and shoulders. It can also help people who lack the courage of their convictions and fail to make decisions, or become overwhelmed by details.

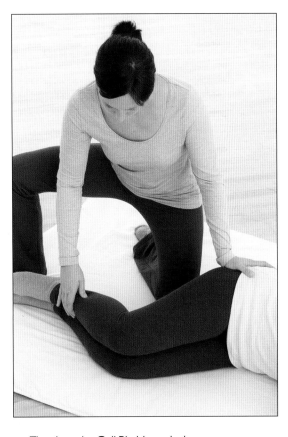

12. Thumbing the Gall Bladder in the leg

After palming, thumb the Channel down to the knee. Below the knee, locate GB 34 (see far left). From here work down toward the ankle, along the bony edge of the fibula. Cross in front of the ankle and thumb down to the space between the 4th and 5th toe. Always consider working the lower GB Channel for acute headaches, eye troubles, insomnia, and irritability.

GB 34

GB 40

The Liver Channel in the lower leg

Work on the Liver Channel affects all areas of the body as it promotes the free flow of Ki. Particular areas of benefit are the lower abdomen, including bowel and bladder function, but especially irregularity and pain of menstruation in women, also the external genitals of both sexes, the chest and ribs, the throat, eyes, and the top of the head. Troubles in any of these areas, especially if they are associated with frustration, depression, sudden outbursts of anger, or any other emotional stress, indicate involvement of the Liver. Stress blocks the Ki causing pain and irregularity.

Completing the routine

After palming and thumbing the Liver Channel, ask your partner to turn briefly to the supine position before moving on to the other side to repeat the whole routine. At the end, work on both feet with your partner again in the supine position (see opposite).

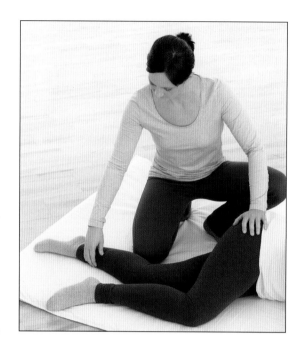

13. Palming and Thumbing the Liver Channel

Palm the Channel along the inside leg, leaning into the relaxed tendon of the upper thigh, down past the knee and on to the calf, then close behind the bone on the lower leg to the ankle. Keep your support hand on the sacral region.

Thumb along the border of the tendon near the groin, along the middle of the inner thigh to the knee. Work into the classical point, Liver 8, in the end of the knee crease.

The Channel runs on down the calf muscle behind the Spleen Channel, but about halfway down, it crosses in front of the Spleen Channel to continue very close behind the edge of the bone, as shown above. Joining the Spleen Channel at Sp 6, "Three-Yin Meeting", it then crosses in front of the ankle, over the top of the foot to the big toe.

Working on the feet

With your partner lying supine you can give special attention at the end of your session to the feet, which have particular significance for the Liver. Both the Liver and Gall Bladder can be upset by rich and spicy foods, stimulant drugs, and alcohol. These, along with the emotions, can combine to overheat the Liver. Its Yang energy then rises forcefully to the head causing acute headaches, sore eyes, dizziness, and nausea. This sounds like a hangover, and it could be, on occasions of excess. But more serious and chronic disharmonies can result in similar symptoms in the long term. Migraines are often a result of the over-stressed lifestyle of busy, creative people who work hard and play hard. Unpredictable moods, irritability, insomnia, red eyes, and indigestion are common symptoms of the Liver on overdrive – called "Liver Fire rising". The last few tsubos on the Liver and Gall Bladder Channels (see p. 141 and opposite) can reduce Liver Fire.

Liver 3 ("Great Pouring")

Working on this point increases the Yin of the Liver – Liver Blood. This nourishes tendons and ligaments, helping all tightness, tension, and spasms. It spreads Liver Ki, reducing pains and obstruction along its Channel and helps regularity and smoothness of all its functions. It eases emotional stress and helps all headaches whether due to excess or weakness.

Liver 2 ("Walk Between")

This is more useful when symptoms are acute, irritating, dry, or hot. It is the "Fire point" of the the Liver Channel. Use it with Liver 3 for bad headaches, period pains, nausea, or painful, difficult urination.

Liv 2

Liv 3

14. Working on the feet

Rotate each foot at the ankle joint, then grasp and stretch each one in turn, first away from the body, leaning back, then toward the head. Press the Liver tsubos calmly and methodically. Hold the feet for a moment to finish.

9. TRADITIONAL DIAGNOSIS

One of the highest goals of Far-Eastern medicine is to help others to live in harmony with the Tao, the Way of Nature. The illnesses that we all experience from time to time are part of this Way. We progress through a series of imbalances, larger or smaller, just as the weather, manifesting the changing seasons, is sometimes rough, violent, unpredictable, but still part of the overall harmony of nature. Our illnesses represent an opportunity to learn about ourselves, and to change and improve our lifestyles. In the West our attempts to banish sickness from our lives ignore the real possibilities for improvement that these illnesses bring.

We mistake the symptoms of an illness for the disease itself. Our medicinal drugs, an armoury of painkillers, antibiotics, anti-inflammatories, anti-histamines, and anti-depressants, with all their attendant side-effects, suppress and confuse the body's clear expression that all is not well inside. Or we may ignore our troubles in the hope that they will go away. Whichever route we take, the constitution has limits: we can only go on like this for so long.

Traditional Oriental medicine relates the events in our bodies to our lives and the environment (see p. 18). It interprets symptoms and signs as a signature of underlying disharmony but accepts these changes as fundamental. Your shiatsu treatment helps to restore balance and harmony in your partner. The traditional causes of disease are described on pages 146–54. Diagnostic methods are discussed on pages 159–61.

For readers of this book it is important to use the information wisely. It is intended to provide guidelines for your work. Use it in the spirit of humility, as a way of understanding your shiatsu partner's immediate needs and as a basis for discussion of lifestyle and the possible causes of illness. If you are not a professional then advise friends to seek help from a skilled practitioner if necessary. Your shiatsu can still be of valuable help.

In the end, once all the different methods are learned and assimilated, diagnosis and treatment merge and become one. The relationship between giver and receiver develops through attentive communication, mutual respect, care, and trust.

THE TRADITIONAL CAUSES OF DISEASE

Understanding the causes of disease helps you interpret the particular symptoms and signs that the body produces as an indication of disharmony. By recognizing the origin of the disharmony, the sick person can make adjustments that will speed recovery and improve his or her health and resistance. This may involve alterations in diet, activities, or attitudes – habitual ways of being in, or relating to, the world. In this way, illness can be used as a catalyst for positive change.

The nine main causes of disease are divided into internal and external categories, plus miscellaneous causes (see right). Each upsets the functions of the Organs and Channels in specific ways (see pp. 147–54). Their effects are either more Yin or more Yang. Emotions, climate, and diet form part of the picture of connections with the Five Elements, as described and illustrated in this section. Refer back to page 22 for the progression of illnesses through the Five Element sequences.

Resistance

The severity of symptoms reflects the strength of the disease relative to the person's resistance, and the degree of struggle between them.

People with a weaker constitution will be susceptible to milder adverse influences. Their symptoms will tend to be mild but more persistent. But if the Ki and Blood are strong, and the mind flourishing, a person will be more adaptable and able to withstand greater extremes.

However, excessive demands of work, emotional stress, poor diet, or climatic exposure may overwhelm or wear down even the strongest individuals. Their illnesses will tend to be more dramatic but mostly short-lived, as they normally recover quickly.

EXTERNAL CAUSES

THE SIX CLIMATIC FACTORS

Heat, Fire, Dryness, Wind, Cold, Damp

INTERNAL CAUSES

THE SEVEN EMOTIONS

Joy, Overthinking, Worry, Sadness, Fear, Fright, Anger

POOR OR INAPPROPRIATE DIET

OVERWORK

EXCESS SEXUAL ACTIVITY

WEAK CONSTITUTION

MISCELLANEOUS CAUSES

Poisoning; insect, snake, and animal bites

Trauma, injury

Wrong treatment

EXTERNAL CAUSES – THE CLIMATIC FACTORS

The weather is the Ki of the outer environment. Our bodies adapt naturally to the climate and normally we can use our common sense to dress according to the prevailing conditions. But sometimes even the mildest change in the weather may catch us unprepared and upset our equilibrium, especially if we are run down and our defences are low. The Yang Channels and the Lungs are the most important lines of defence.

The impact of the weather is acknowledged in much Oriental art, as in this woodblock print by Hiroshige.

The Effect of Climate on Body

Climatic excess	Symptoms and associations	Element	Channels and Organs affected
Heat and Fire	High temperature, fever, thirst, red face, and skin rashes, profuse sweating, fear of heat, irritability, restlessness. Extreme Heat invades the Pericardium causing delerium and collapse (as in sunstroke).	Fire	Heart Small Intestine Triple Burner Pericardium
Dryness	Similar to Heat but milder. Prolonged Heat or fever — dry Large Intestine: dry skin, lips, and throat, constipation; dry Stomach: nausea and dry mouth; dry indoor heating or warm, dry wind — Lungs: dry cough.	Metal	Large Intestine Lungs
Wind	The most vicious climatic excess; it drives other influences into the body; unpredictable, sudden, and violent symptoms come and go, and move about. Headaches, stuffy or streaming nose, sneezing, stiff neck, dizziness, itching, spasms, tics, and fear of wind.	Wood	Gall Bladder Liver
Cold	Fevers — the main symptoms are chills, shivering, little or no sweating, and fear of cold. Cold causes contraction and blocks the flow of Ki: cramps, spasms, and fixed pains in the joints. Cold affects the Water element: profuse, pale urination, pain, watery colds, and feeling chilled to the bone.	Water	Bladder Kidneys
Damp	Damp housing conditions, sitting or sleeping on damp ground, as well as prolonged damp weather produce symptoms that are sluggish in onset and are difficult and slow to cure. They often affect the lower body and limbs: swelling, numbness, feelings of heaviness, stiff, swollen joints, tiredness, and sometimes a dull, heavy headache. Internally Damp attacks the Spleen: phlegm, excessive mucus, and discharges.	Earth	Stomach Spleen

The Yang Channels

Yang protects the outside; Yin nourishes the inside. The Yang Channels circulate the outer and upper parts of the body and play a role in defence generally. Climatic excesses usually affect the upper part of the body (except for Damp, which often rises from the earth and affects the joints in the lower body). Therefore acute disease caused by the weather is often best treated by the Yang Channels.

The Lungs

External factors and acute illness do not usually affect the Yin Organs directly, but the Lungs are an exception. They are situated highest in the body like a protective "lid" and open to the exterior. They are the most Yang of the Yin Organs.

The Lungs circulate "Protective Ki", which fights the invading influence. Frequent coughs, colds, or fevers are a sign of weak Lungs and Protective Ki.

Internal correspondences

A Yin–Yang disharmony within the body, when associated with weak functioning of the Organs, may produce symptoms very similar to the external climates. Because of this, they are referred to as interior Damp, interior Wind, and so on. These conditions affect the Yin Organs as often as the Yang.

INTERNAL CAUSES – THE SEVEN EMOTIONS

Your emotions enable you to communicate your deep feelings. If they are repressed, the emotions persist and may become unbalanced.

Oriental medicine associates the emotions with the Yin Organs at the core of your being. Each Organ is connected with a particular emotion (see the Five Element Chart, p. 21), but two Organs bear the brunt of all emotional difficulties – the Heart and Liver. Treating the appropriate Organs along their Channels can support people through emotionally stressful times, helping to regulate imbalances, and prevent fur ther upset. The close, supportive contact that shiatsu offers can be invaluable in times of stress.

Emotions and the Heart and Liver

The Heart is associated with love, warmth, and the formation of relationships. It houses the Mind, or Spirit, which governs general stability. Emotional stress and shock can lead to mental disturbance, anxiety, and unstable behaviour.

The Liver governs the free flow of Ki, which relates to our expression of feelings. The repression of any emotion restrains the Liver and blocks Ki. This can cause obstruction or pain anywhere in the body, a sense of stuffiness in the chest or diaphragm area as well as depression or forceful explosions of feeling (see "Anger" opposite).

THE SEVEN EMOTIONS

Joy

This is the emotion of the Heart. It calms the Mind and relaxes the Ki. The Heart's "ambassador", the Pericardium, brings joy and happiness to the Heart by mediating and regulating relationships. Excessive stimulation of the senses or passionate over-indulgence in excitement and pleasure are said to distract and unsettle the Mind and disturb the Heart, causing its Fire to flare up. Over-exuberance suggests a Heart imbalance.

Sadness or grief

Sadness results from disappointment, or more seriously from separation and loss. It is said to "dissolve" the Ki and principally affects the Lungs, expressed in its "sound" — weeping (see p. 21). Sadness is felt in the Heart and affects the whole chest, producing heaviness, breathlessness, tiredness, and depression. We need time to express our sadness or grief; rituals for dealing with change and loss probably help us to cope better with these emotions.

Worry

Worry springs from insecurity and tends to deplete the Spleen, which belongs to the Earth element and which in turn relates to support, nourishment, and early nurture. Worry "knots" the Ki of the Lungs, tightening the chest and shoulders and constricting breathing. We can feel immobilized by worry. The Lungs and the Spleen are the sources of

the body's True Ki, so worry depletes Ki generally.

Pensiveness

This emotion is similar to worry but relates specifically to our capacity for mental work. The Spleen governs the intellect and so can suffer from the effects of overthinking, made worse by lack of exercise and irregular meals. The results are weakness, indigestion, and phlegm.

A weak Spleen can manifest as obsession with order and detail — the making of endless lists, calorie counting etc. Also, when, as computer users, we become "hooked to our screens", the Spleen's Ki is compromised.

Fear

Fear is associated with the Kidneys. It makes Ki descend and affects the "pit of the Stomach".

In children it can manifest as night fears and bed-wetting. Adults with Kidney deficiency and weak constitutions may also be prone to "irrational" fears and anxiety, insomnia, spontaneous sweating, and dry mouth.

Unacceptable fear is sometimes unconsciously transferred into a strong drive to undertake dangerous occupations or pastimes, which justify the confrontation of fear. But if the root of the fear is not recognized, Kidney Yang can deplete the Yin, causing "uprising Fire" problems in the Liver and Heart.

Fright

This emotion is similar to fear but more extreme. It is identical to shock, associated with physical or emotional trauma. It suspends or scatters the Ki and affects the Kidneys and the Heart. The Kidneys store Ki for defence and may be suddenly drained. The Heart suffers from disruption of the Mind. Shock is characterized by loss of memory, disorientation, palpitations, dizziness, trembling, sweating, and fainting. Unresolved shock ties up the energy, which causes depletion.

Anger

This is the emotion of the Liver. It can take several modified forms, including irritability, frustration, jealousy, and rage. Anger makes the Ki rise, and with it the bile. A bitter taste in the mouth, red or yellowish eyes, redness of the face and neck, dizziness, and especially headaches are symptoms and signs of "rebellious" Liver Ki.

If suppressed, the Yang dynamic of anger turns into the Yin state of depression, which causes stagnation of Liver Ki and aches, pains, and feelings of oppression, stuffiness, or bloatedness. Either form of Liver emotion can upset the Stomach and Spleen. Its Wood energy expands and then "invades" the Earth Organs (see p. 21) causing nausea, acidity, vomiting, or diarrhoea.

Constitution

Life begins at conception. In the womb the fetus is nourished by "Prenatal Ki", the foundation of the constitution, stored in the Kidneys in the form of Essence. The parents' health, especially that of the mother during pregnancy, and the circumstances of birth establish initial constitutional strength and determine the amount of Prenatal Ki. This is supplemented after birth by Postnatal Ki from air and food. Serious illnesses or accidents may weaken constitutional Ki. It may also be squandered by careless living. However, careful diet and avoidance of extremes conserves it. Teachers of internal exercise systems such as Chi Kung or Tai Chi claim that these increase constitutional reserves.

A weak constitution renders a person more susceptible to illness and this weakness can be a specific cause of Kidney disease.

Excess sex and overwork

The Kidneys are most affected by these two causes of disease, which can be considered together as they can sometimes complicate each other.

Kidney Essence forms the sexual fluids and reproductive substances of both sexes. Kidney Yang provides the energy for sex. The Kidneys are associated with physical drive, including the ability to cope with energetic work. Hard physical work, lifting and bending, or jobs that involve standing for long periods can deplete them. Overdemanding mental work depletes the Spleen as well as the Kidneys.

"Excessive sex" requires common sense in its interpretation. It depends on age, constitutional strength, and circumstance. Traditionally, men deplete their Essence through ejaculation, but excessive orgasm weakens the Kidneys in both sexes. Too many late nights, sex while drunk, or when tired from overwork can all be contributory factors.

Women lose less of their sexual fluids during sex and so tend to recover more quickly, but they can suffer from the physical demands of pregnancy, which also depletes the Essence. Childbirth, feeding, and caring for young children also make great demands.

Miscellaneous causes

These include bites and poisons, trauma, epidemics, and wrong treatment. Wrong treatment is as prevalent today as it has ever been. Illnesses that are caused by wrong treatment are known as iatrogenic diseases.

Diet

Our technological advances have led us down the path of consuming processed, de-natured, reconstructed, additive-laced foods that generally lower health and resistance to disease. The proliferation of dietary theories, books, special regimes, food substitutes, and supplements confuses most people, and produces a dependency on special products and "expert" advice. In the face of this, traditional Chinese medicine offers a refreshing down-to-earth approach to diet, advocating balance, moderation, and common sense.

The balance of Yin and Yang in food is shown in the chart overleaf. The foods in the central area of the chart are more balanced than those at the top and bottom. But even the extreme foods can be eaten and enjoyed in moderation. Our diet can create problems if we eat mostly Yin or mostly Yang foods; so can habitually eating our meals too fast, or eating while angry, anxious, or under stress, late in the day, or at irregular times. Eat regularly, chew slowly and allow time for digestion. In this way all kinds of foods can be tolerated.

Five Element theory categorizes foods according to flavour, listing "five tastes" associated with the Five Elements (see chart overleaf below). A little of each flavour nourishes its associated Yin Organ but excesses unbalance the cycle, causing trouble in any related Organs. Cravings are manifestations of imbalance.

Yin and Yang influence in foods

Rich, spicy and hot foods increase Yang in the body. They put stress on the Liver, aggravate "hot" illnesses and create phlegm.

Cold, fresh, and raw foods put stress on the Spleen. Too many Yin foods aggravate "cold" conditions with poor circulation, weak digestion with loose bowels, and damp, watery, or phlegmy illnesses. Consult and study the chart on the right.

greasy fried food   chilli pepper   black pepper
red wine and spirits   cinnamon   coffee
lamb   garlic   ginger

YANG EXTREME   white wine and aperitifs
baked and roasted foods
peaches   cooked whole grains, flakes

beef   chicken   grapes   rice   peas
corn
beans

root vegetables   oats
potatoes

dates, raisins   wheat
honey
millet   leafy vegetables
nuts and seeds
barley

celery   asparagus
buckwheat   milk
eggs   flours, bread, pasta   apples   fruit juices

herbal teas   white fish   pork   pears   beers
boiled foods   raw foods   water   mineral waters

YIN EXTREME
iced drinks   sugary drinks   colas
salt   seaweeds and shellfish
tomato   melon   banana   cucumber
lettuce
ice cream   cold, raw foods

Five Element flavour associations

ELEMENT	Earth	Metal	Water	Wood	Fire
ORGAN	Spleen	Lung	Kidney	Liver	Heart
FLAVOUR	Sweet	Pungent	Salty	Sour	Bitter

TRADITIONAL ORIENTAL DIAGNOSIS

A practitioner takes note of a patient's constitution, disposition, history, and lifestyle as well as any obvious symptoms in making a diagnosis. The four traditional methods used to obtain this information are looking, asking, listening and smelling, and touching (see p. 157). No one method can supply a diagnosis and quick judgements or fixed interpretations are best avoided. Each method adds valuable insights from which a pattern emerges.

Familiarity with the organs and Channels and their inter-related functions (as described in Part Two) will help you understand the particular pattern of disharmony in your partner and guide your own approach to treatment.

Looking

The general build, posture, and way of moving gives us insight into a person's constitutional vitality and attitude to life. A thin, wiry person will tend toward overactive Yang Ki, which can lead to exhaustion. Heavier, obese people may have weaker Ki and suffer from poor circulation and digestion. Imbalances in a person's build, muscular tension or strain in posture reveal compensating or defensive investment of Ki in one part of the body related to weakness in another part (see pp. 158–59).

More detailed observation of the skin, face (see following pages), eyes, tongue, and other parts of the body also form an important part of traditional diagnosis.

Facial diagnosis

Head hair indicates a Kidney condition. Premature balding or greying shows deficient Kidneys.

Sheen of hair reflects the health of the Lungs. Dry or brittle hair indicates weak Lungs.

Deep frown lines may indicate a temperamental Liverish disposition/constitution.

The brightness of the eyes relates to the Mind and Essence – the constitutional strength of Heart and Kidneys. If the eyes shine the person has "good spirit" and can recover even from a serious disease.

The colour of the upper lid relates to Spleen; lower lid to Stomach.

The whites of the eyes reflect the Lungs. Red indicates dryness and Heat. Yellow indicates phlegm.

Dark swellings under eyes result from weak Kidneys.

The colour of the corners of the eye relate to the Heart, red means Heat; pale means weak Blood.

The colour of the upper cheek relates to the Heart and the Fire element. Puffy upper cheeks indicate a weak Small Intestine.

The iris and whole eye is part of the Liver function. Red eyes mean Liver Heat. Other eye troubles suggest a weak Liver.

The colour of the lower cheek relates to the Lungs and the Metal element. Sagging lines or puffiness suggest a weak Large Intestine.

Ear lobe indicates the constitution and strength of Kidneys. Long and full ear lobes are a mark of strength and vice versa.

The colour of the tip of the nose is a Spleen indicator.

Bridge of nose area can reveal Liver and Gall Bladder disorders.

Lips and mouth are part of Stomach and Spleen function. Dry red lips and bleeding gums indicate Stomach Heat. Pale lips are the result of weak Spleen or weak Blood.

A short chin indicates constitutionally weak Kidneys. A strong chin suggests a strong constitution.

The teeth are part of the Kidney function. Weak, loose, or "dry" teeth suggests a Kidney deficiency.

Facial diagnosis

Facial diagnosis is widely practised in the Orient by doctors and fortune tellers alike. Many different systems and interpretations have developed since classical times and this can easily confuse the beginner. Only the most commonly accepted aspects are given here (see opposite).

The colours of the complexion give a general guide to the condition of the body. Red indicates overactive Yang or Heat, while pale or white areas show weak Ki and Blood, poor circulation, and Cold. A bright or shiny complexion shows a Yang condition. This is less serious than a Yin depletion indicated by dull, dry or lifeless colouration. For the relationship between the colour of the areas of the face and the Five Elements, see the chart on p. 21.

Asking

Straightforward, attentive inquiry after the details of a person's condition is an important diagnostic method. Begin with the onset and duration of any current problems and the person's general health and history. Then ask about the location of any pain or other symptoms that may indicate which Organs and Channels are involved. Ask about feelings of cold, heat, or feverishness and find out if the person is tired and lethargic, or nervous and restless. This indicates the balance of Yin and Yang as well as the overall energy levels. Other details, ranging from appetite, digestion, and excretions, to mood, occupation, and lifestyle help us to picture the disharmony.

Listening and smelling

Listening and smelling constitute one method in traditional diagnosis. The strength of the voice relates to the Lungs and indicates the strength of a person's Ki. The Heart and Mind influence coherence of speech. Wheezy breathing indicates phlegm (Damp), while quick, shallow breaths slow depletion of Heart and Lung Ki. The sound of a cough tells us whether the Lungs are affected by Dryness or Damp.

The "Five Sounds" of the Five Element chart (see p. 21) relate to the expression of emotion as well as a quality of voice.

Subtle body odours are not easy to interpret. At the the most simple level, a strong smell from perspiration or other excretions indicates a "Hot" disease.

Touching

The practice of shiatsu naturally places a strong emphasis on diagnosis through touch. Feeling for tsubos and learning to "listen" with your hands are dealt with throughout this book. You can obtain more information about your partner by feeling and pressing various parts of the body for comparison, examining the Channels and areas of pain for differences of temperature, resistance, and reaction (see pp. 158–59). Even more important is feeling the subtle qualities of the abdomen, or Hara. In Chinese medicine pulse diagnosis is the most important and profound diagnostic tool, but the Japanese have also developed Hara diagnosis to a refined level. Basic Hara diagnosis is introduced later in the chapter (pp. 160–61).

TOUCH DIAGNOSIS – KYO AND JITSU

Stresses from the outside and within the body create distortions of Ki in the Channels. Distortions are always present to some degree as a result of the day-to-day demands of life on the organism.

Two Japanese terms, "kyo" and "jitsu", express the dynamics of this process. Kyo is the primary distortion, an internal "need". Jitsu is the compensating response that seeks to fill the need. For example, when you feel hungry (kyo) you make yourself a meal (jitsu) to satisfy your hunger or, on the autonomic level, when you feel the cold (kyo), your skin contracts (jitsu) to form goose-bumps.

When the needs of a kyo condition cannot be met, the body becomes vulnerable and secondary kyo–jitsu patterns develop over the earlier ones. We call this illness, but all organisms have defensive and compensating strategies that involve a shift in energy, in an effort to restore harmony.

There will be changes in the quality of the body tissues – tenderness or numbness, muscle tension or flaccidity, stiffness or looseness in the joints, and so on – with more subtle alterations in the flow of Ki in the Channels. Practise feeling the difference between kyo and jitsu conditions in your partner, and treat according to the principles outlined on these pages.

Kyo and Jitsu

Masunaga explained kyo and jitsu by using the example of single-celled organisms.
Their growth, maturity, and reproduction creates an inner need for energy and produces corresponding distortions at the surface. For example, an organism that has increasing need (right) invests energy at the border in order to propel itself toward food (centre) which it then engulfs and assimilates, returning temporarily to a state of relative equilibrium (far right).

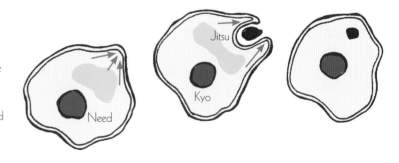

Kyo and jitsu in the Channels

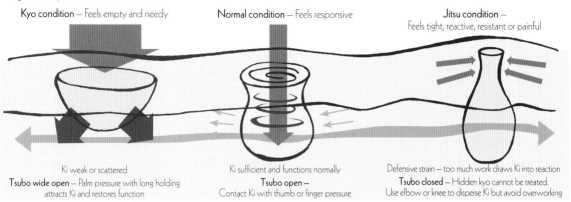

Kyo condition — Feels empty and needy

Normal condition — Feels responsive

Jitsu condition — Feels tight, reactive, resistant or painful

Ki weak or scattered
Tsubo wide open — Palm pressure with long holding attracts Ki and restores function

Ki sufficient and functions normally
Tsubo open —
Contact Ki with thumb or finger pressure

Defensive strain — too much work draws Ki into reaction
Tsubo closed — Hidden kyo cannot be treated.
Use elbow or knee to disperse Ki but avoid overworking

Kyo and jitsu in acute illness

A person's constitution may be strong enough to "fight off" an invading influence or compensate for disturbed function, but it can be helpful in acute cases to "sedate" or "disperse" jitsu areas or Channels. Apply strong pressure for a short duration. Traditional points can also be stimulated in this way. Their specific action on the Ki guides or prompts the healing process.

Remember that there will be a corresponding kyo aspect needing attention and support. The body's reserves may be depleted and the person will also need time to recover.

Kyo and jitsu in chronic illness

If distortions persist on a deeper level, chronic illness may develop, with both kyo and jitsu aspects. Kyo is the underlying Yin aspect, the root of the disharmony. There may be blocked emotions, internal weaknesses or underfunctioning Organs, with a corresponding stiffness, flaccidity, or emptiness in related Channels. Jitsu, the Yang aspect, is like a messenger, manifesting as tension, pain, or other reactive symptoms.

These jistu aspects will attract your attention and you may be tempted to "treat" them (for example massage tight or painful areas). But they are simply pointing to the root of the disharmony.

The most effective shiatsu treats the primary kyo aspects of the energetic distortion with supportive and penetrating pressure on kyo Channels and tsubos. This directly addresses the inner need, bringing Ki and Blood to tonify deficient areas and releasing Ki from both deeply held blockage and compensating jitsu patterns.

Chinese laws of diagnosis

The applications of kyo and jitsu suggested here are a simplification of classical Chinese laws of diagnosis and treatment. These recognize, firstly, that illness occurs at different depths in the body; secondly, that you should find out and treat the root of disease rather than its manifesting symptoms. Thirdly, as a rule, you should tonify kyo conditions – inner deficiencies of Ki and Blood – as a priority over dispersing excesses and blockages.

FOCUSING ON THE HARA

Hara diagnosis is used in Japan as an aspect of touch diagnosis. As with pulse, tongue, or facial diagnosis (see p. 156), it takes much practice to perfect.

Hara work reveals useful information about the condition of the receiver. As your touch becomes more sensitive and your understanding develops, you will learn to interpret what you feel in terms of kyo–jitsu. But always retain an open, or "beginner's" mind; otherwise you will only pick up a reflection of your preconceptions.

All your shiatsu treatments will produce changes in the Hara. You can monitor changes in your partner by feeling the condition of the Hara before and after treatment, also noting

changes over time, between treatments. Sitting by your partner's side to work with the Hara, you have the chance to combine all the other methods of diagnosis – looking, asking, and listening, with your touch. The essence of good treatment is a feeling of communication and empathy "Hara to Hara".

Palpating the Hara

To palpate the Hara, keep your fingers extended but relaxed, and use perpendicular pressure of your relaxed arm. No further leaning is necessary. Don't push or press. Encourage your partner to relax, heed their breathing, and "listen" with your fingers.

Simple Hara diagnosis

Simple Hara diagnosis distinguishes two main regions of the Hara, the upper and the lower. The upper region, between the ribs and the navel, should feel soft, flexible, but lively. The lower region, below the navel and including the pubic region, should feel firm and strong. Another interpretation of the Hara regions divides them in the same way as the Triple Burner (see below). Masunaga developed a refinement (see below right) which offers more detail – there is a zone for each meridian. Other methods were based on the "five elements". Practise the simple approach unless you have a teacher versed in a specific method.

Learning from the Hara

By gently feeling the Hara, you can obtain information about the Organs and Channels, using the guidance on the facing page. To interpret what you feel, you will need to develop your sense of kyo and jitsu qualities (see pp. 158–59). Jitsu is reactive, energetic, lively, tight and sometimes warm. Kyo is soft, flaccid, weak, passive and sometimes cold or stiff. Try to develop an unobtrusive approach to working on this region. Your partner may feel protective about the area, but by your actions will be reassured.

The upper region controls circulation and transmits the Ki (Breath) downwards to the Kidneys. This area should feel supple, soft, and unconstrained.

Around the navel should feel lively, flexible, and responsive, neither hard nor soggy.

The Tanden is associated with the Kidneys and source Ki. It "receives and stores" and should feel firm and strong.

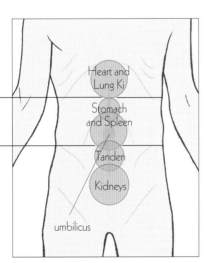

Hara diagnosis, following the "Triple Burner" regions

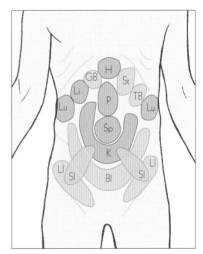

Hara diagnosis following Masunaga's arrangement

A PRACTICE ROUTINE
THE BREATH, THE CHEST & THE HARA

Hara diagnosis depends on the breath reaching the Tanden. If tension blocks the movement of the ribs and diaphragm the breath is shallow and restricted, and Ki from the lungs will not circulate or descend. The function of the Hara as a vital centre will be limited and so diagnosis will be difficult or impossible.

Hara work provides a focus for self-awareness and change in the receiver while helping you, the giver, to integrate your shiatsu routines. Aware of limitations, you can develop your skill and sensitivity gradually, noting the changes in breathing and kyo–jitsu qualities in the Hara.

The Chest and Hara routine
Keeling next to your partner, take a few moments to tune in to your own state and relax with your feelings, otherwise your interpretation of your partner's condition will be coloured and confused by your own. Observe your partner's facial expression, the way the shoulders are held, the depth and rhythm of the breathing and any tightness in the diaphragm.

As an exercise, try treating the three Yin Channels in the arm, which strongly influence the breath and emotional energy. You can treat them all with your partner in the supine position. The illustrations below will remind you of the arm positions that open each Channel most readily for your work. While practising this sequence you will be able to feel the subtle relationship between breath and Hara.

1. Making contact — Hara and lower back
Rest your near hand, palm down, on your partner's Hara, with the heel of your hand below the navel and your fingers above. Relax your shoulder and elbow. Initially, just slide your other hand gently under the arch of your partner's back. The tighter the muscles, the more arched the lumbar region will be. Note the general tonal quality and how the breath moves in the Hara.

162

2. Checking the Hara areas

Then, bring your hand from the back to support the upper Hara. With your near hand, gently probe the abdomen above and then below the navel with your fingers extended. Practise describing to yourself mentally the different qualities that you feel.

3. Arm rotation supporting the shoulder

Changing position, pick up the wrist and support your partner's shoulder to perform one or two full arm rotations in preparation for shiatsu along each of the three Yin Channels in the arm. First treat the Lung Channel (see p. 80).

4. Treating the Pericardium Channel

For the Pericardium, position the arm further out to the side, palm uppermost. Lean down on to the front of the shoulder with your supporting hand. Palm and thumb the Channel with the other – directly through the centre of the biceps muscle and down the middle of the lower arm.

5. Treating the Heart Channel

Lift and stretch the arm once more and replace it, folding it gently back. If your partner's shoulder is tight, do not force the arm too far. Let it drop back out again slightly so that the arm rests firmly on the ground. Then you can lean your body weight with confidence to palm and thumb the Heart Channel, along the inner edge of the biceps muscle through the crook of the elbow, along to the wrist and little finger. Your mother (resting) hand can support at Heart 1 in the centre of the armpit. Replace the arm in a comfortable position. Repeat the work on the other arm and replace it by the receiver's side. Finish by leaning on your partner's shoulders for a few moments (see p. 91), then check the Hara again for changes in the kyo–jitsu pattern.

10. EVERYDAY SHIATSU

As you become familiar with the shiatsu routines that are demonstrated in Chapters 4, 6, 7, and 8, you will gain the confidence to adapt the routines to suit the particular needs of your partner. Having learned the basic techniques and Channel pathways, you can adopt a more versatile approach in your shiatsu sessions. This chapter explores some of the ways in which you can use your knowledge of the Channels to develop routines for particular ailments or for the circumstances of everyday life.

The short routine for the head and feet given on pages 166–71 is suitable for treating people who are tired over-stressed, and who cannot relax or sleep well. It is relaxing for the giver as well as the receiver, and can be done at the end of a busy day. Young children and pregnant women can also benefit from shiatsu treatment: follow the routines adapted to their special requirements on pages 172–75.

For those people who are uncomfortable lying on their front, or those who are not happy lying down at all, try the routine for shiatsu in the sitting position (see pp. 176–83). Use this for giving shiatsu to an elderly relative, or for treating a friend with asthma, or a colleague with a headache while you are at work. Each of these may prefer to sit either on the floor or in a chair.

Try to follow the principles of advanced technique, sometimes known as the "inner" principles (see pp. 50–53), and you will be able to adapt your shiatsu sessions to working on your partner in the sitting position and to any of the other demonstrations in this chapter.

Knowing how to adapt your shiatsu sessions not only helps you work with greater confidence but it develops an easy way with touch that positively enhances the richness and quality of your life.

Rotating the arm in preparation for shiatsu on the neck and shoulders.

SHIATSU FOR THE HEAD & FEET

When people are tired, tense, agitated, and unable to relax, they are manifesting a Yin–Yang disharmony. If Yin becomes too weak to attract and hold the Yang, or Yang becomes too strong in the body, the Yang separates and "rebels" upward. Headaches, nervousness, irritability, restlessness, insomnia, dryness of the eyes, nose, or throat, thirst, hot feelings in the chest or head, and flushed cheeks are typical symptoms of this kind of imbalance. Giving

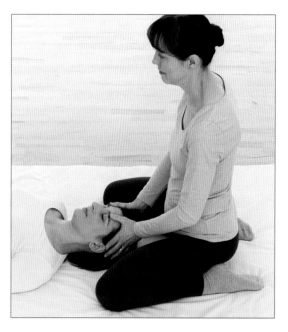

1. Holding the head

Before you start to give pressure to the tsubos, just calmly hold the head for a moment. Rest your thumbs flat across the forehead and hold your palms and fingers over the temples.

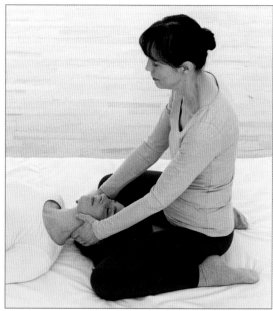

2. Stretching the spine

Use a low pillow for this routine. Sit at your partner's head, relax and lean on their shoulders. Move your hands under the neck, overlap your fingers and, with your hands against the base of the skull, lift up and lean back with your entire body to open and stretch the spine. Replace your partner's head, straightening the neck by pulling the neck and head back toward you.

shiatsu to the head and feet is often helpful in these circumstances. The routine lasts only 15 or 20 minutes. Try it at the end of a working day, or just before bed time, when its benefits will be most useful.

Begin with the head to disperse the Yang Ki and help it descend. Then work at the feet to strengthen the Yin, which attracts the Yang down. The Yin ascends to calm the Mind, cool the head, and moisten the eyes and throat. It helps the eyes to close at night.

The role of Yin and Yang

Yin attracts Yang; Yang attracts Yin. Yang is active and protects Yin; Yin nourishes and supports Yang. Yang is warm and drying; Yin is cool and moistening. Yang Ki regulates the sensory "openings". The Yin Channels carry nourishment and moisture upward to the sensory orifices.

3. Working on the face

Start by working on both sides of the face at once. The symmetry of your thumb pressure will feel quite appropriate and comfortable as long as you maintain support with your extended fingers at the side of your partner's head. Use your thumbs to follow the Bladder Channel up over the forehead from the inner corner of the eyebrow (Bl 2) toward the top of the head. Next, follow the inner line of the Gall Bladder Channel from GB 14 up and over the head. Then, using one thumb over the other, follow the Governing Channel from "Seal Hall", the point between the eyebrows, up to the top of the head.

It is not necessary to follow the Channels rigorously. Try working along the eyebrow line; then follow the contours of the face, below the eyes and across and under the cheek bones. Finally, work round the line of the jawbone, using the thumbs on top and curling the fingers under the chin. Any tsubos that you find relate to the Yang Channels on the face (see pp. 70–71); but there may be some classical points that you feel will be particularly useful for your partner. Feel free to concentrate on them as you come to them.

"Seal Hall"
"Fish Spine"
GB14
Bl 2
TB 23
Bl 1
GB 1
St 2
St 3
LI 20
SI 18
GV 26
"Middle of Person"

4. The eyes

Work with the thumb is sometimes difficult; use the little finger for Bl 1, "Eye Brightness", which also helps insomnia. This point is 1/10 in (0.25 cm) above the inner corner of the eye. Press inward and upward.

Points around the eye socket are particularly useful for eye problems. Some also help in nose and sinus trouble and most relieve headaches, too. These are annotated in the diagram on p. 167 and include "Fish Spine", located in the middle of each eyebrow; "Seal Hall", between the brows on the mid line Channel; and GB 14, "Yang White", 1 in (2.5 cm) above "Fish Spine", which marks the beginning of the inner line of the Gall Bladder Channel over the head.

5. Working on the side of the head and the base of the skull

After working over the face turn the head a little to the side, rolling it into your palm for support. Now work down the side of the head, first thumbing the Stomach Channel from the corner of the forehead down in front of the ear to the muscle at the corner of the jaw. Then systematically work the tsubos along and within the hairline and around the ear. Finish by finding the tsubos under the base of the skull (see left). Feel for any hollows where your pressure feels accepted. Some of these are classical points with known benefits for the eyes, ears, and other sense organs. Some also calm the Mind and so are useful for insomnia, nervousness, or irritability.

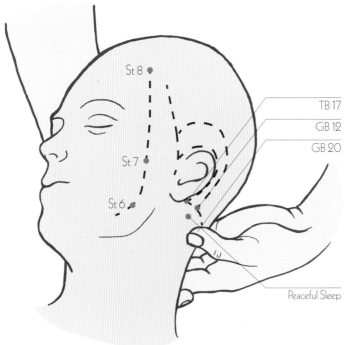

St 8

St 7

St 6

TB 17

GB 12

GB 20

Peaceful Sleep

Three-way stretch

This helps loosen and balance the neck. Roll your partner's head from side to side to feel for any resistance. If each side feels the same, begin on either side; otherwise, stretch the easy (kyo) side first (see p. 158).

6. Three-way stretch

Roll the head to face right, lean on the left shoulder with your right hand, and bring your left palm across to the side of the head (see above left). Stretch the neck by leaning gradually into your hands, elbows relaxed, then release. Reach your left hand behind the head to lift and turn it a little further (see above centre). Stretch and release. Then allow the head to roll back on to your palm, and stretch again (see above right). Release. Repeat on the other side.

7. Working on the base of the skull

Roll the head to the centre. Curl your fingers under the base of the skull and pull back slightly for a few moments, supporting the sides of the head with your palms. Then let your fingers find another position, penetrating the softer tissues or hollows (tsubos), and pull back again. Repeat this 2 or 3 times, allowing your partner to adjust, breathe, and relax each time. Then gently break contact and move to the feet.

Treating the feet

Many of us spend much of the day on our feet. "Taking the weight off our feet" or "putting our feet up" are powerful metaphors for relaxation, and relaxation enhances their practical benefits. To work at someone's feet is also a true metaphor for the humble service we offer.

Work on the feet can affect the whole body, harmonizing Yin and Yang via the Channels as described already (see p. 167). The recently rediscovered system of reflexology confirms the ancient Chinese understanding that each part reflects and affects the whole. Troubles of the feet and ankles, such as cramps, rheumatic pains, the effects of sprain, and other injuries can also be treated by careful shiatsu around the affected area and to nearby tsubos.

8. Rotating the ankle

Kneel by your partner's feet and take one foot on to your thigh. Hold the ankle just above the joint. Rotate the foot slowly and firmly with the other hand, a few times in each direction. Steady your arm against your other leg (see above), and work with body movement, not muscle power.

If your partner is relaxed, you should see a slight movement as a visible wave through the body as far as the shoulders and neck, which confirms the improved Ki flow between the head and feet.

9. Thumbing the Yin Channels on the foot

Thumb the Yin Channels on the feet — the Kidney, Spleen, and Liver Channels. Work from the ankle and heel along the inner aspect of the foot. Cross under the arch to the sole for the Kidney Channel and follow the other two to the inner and outer edges of the big toe. Grip and rotate the toe. Give stationary pressure to any tsubos that seem open or responsive.

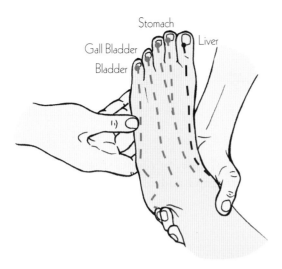

Stomach

Gall Bladder
Liver

Bladder

10. Thumbing the Bladder Channel on the foot

Change hands to work on the Yang Channels on the outer aspect of the foot. Begin with the Bladder Channel and work round the ankle and along the edge of the foot to the small toe. Then work the other Channels from the ankle points to the toes, feeling for the hollows between the bones and tendons. The Gall Bladder Channel goes to the 4th toe; the Stomach Channel has two branches, the main one going to the 2nd toe and another going to the 3rd toe, so work between all the bones.

11. Stretching and rotating the toes

Finish by stretching and rotating all the toes.

Note:

The feet hold much tension and some people are quite sensitive about their feet. The effects of foot shiatsu can be powerfully releasing. Always be prepared to moderate your techniques and routines. Let your partner be your guide.

12. Stretching the foot

Finally, bend and stretch the whole foot in both directions, away from you by using your body weight to lean forward and bend the foot and toes back, then down, by grasping the top of the foot, as shown, and leaning back. Change sides and repeat all the techniques on the other foot.

SHIATSU FOR CHILDREN

Shiatsu with children can be formal or informal, a ritual at bedtime, or useful at any time. Children of all ages can benefit from shiatsu; and so, too, can parents. Shiatsu can literally help parents and children keep in touch with each other during the many phases of their developing relationship.

It is not only an effective means of dealing with children's common minor ailments but a valuable way of reassuring them during illness, expressing feelings of commitment, and helping them to have trust in you. In many Oriental countries, children are encouraged to give massage to their parents when the day's work is finished. The children's valued contribution is a reminder of the reciprocal nature of family relationships.

On the whole, children are more Yang. They are prone to feverish or hot complaints, but their illnesses come and go quickly. They are sensitive and their Ki responds easily to pressure on the Channels and points.

Common ailments

In fevers stroke repeatedly down the spine, also down the Heart Channel to the small finger, and out from the bridge of the nose to the sides of the forehead. For poor digestion, often associated with teething troubles, give circular massage to the abdomen, and massage the thumb and forefinger, especially LI 4. Then massage St 36 and the Stomach line on the foot. For diarrhoea stroke up the Lung and Large Intestine Channels and massage repeatedly up the sacrum; for constipation massage down the sacrum. If the child is restless, irritable, or upset and panicky, try slow, steady massage of the palm, then grasp and gently squeeze along each finger to the fingernail. For bed-wetting and night fears rub the lumbar region to warm the Mei Mon. Hold the Hara and massage Kidney and Bladder points around the ankles.

Massage for under-fives

For very young children (up to five years), rubbing or stroking along the Channels can be more appropriate and effective than pressure. Sometimes a combination of methods works well. Follow the general rule that you should massage away from the centre and down the limbs when the child is strong and fractious, or feverish and restless, with a loud cry or cough. When a child is weak, listless, or nervous, massage up the limbs and toward the centre. Refer to the back of this book for further reading on the natural treatment of children's ailments.

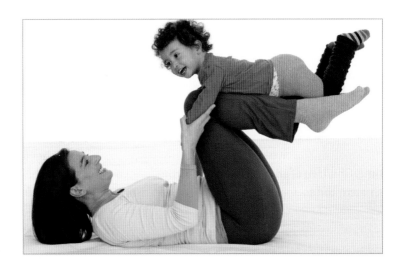

Shiatsu for children

A stroking massage for the chest (see below) – outward for an acute cough, inward from the ribs if the chest is weakened.

SHIATSU FOR PREGNANCY

During pregnancy, a woman's body adapts to the new demands of nourishing and carrying the developing fetus. The mother's Kidney Ki and Essence are the principal sources of nourishment for the child growing within. The Kidneys are the root of Yin and Yang; typical symptoms in pregnancy are associated with the temporary loss of balance due to this diversion of Kidney energies. If the women's constitution is weak, or if she is obliged to continue with strenuous work without sufficient rest, then the Kidneys (and hence other Organs), will be stressed, and symptoms may become persistent or serious.

Exercise, proper diet, and rest are all important. Shiatsu can be a great help, especially in the early and later stages of pregnancy, as discussed below.

Treatment for morning sickness

The Bladder Channel affords a very balanced treatment in pregnancy: it helps the Kidneys and influences all the other Organs via their "associated points" (see p. 121). Concentrate on the middle region near the points for Liver, Gall Bladder, Spleen, and Stomach. Then give particular attention to the Pericardium Channel. Point P 6 is good for all sickness. On the Stomach Channel, work on St 36 and St 44. Lastly, give steady pressure to Liv 3.

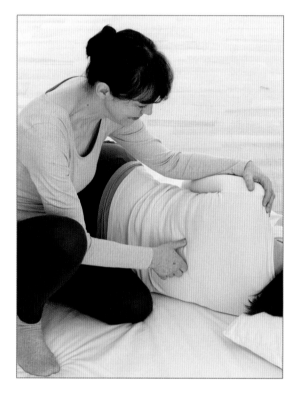

Working the Bladder Channel for morning sickness

Morning sickness, caused by "rebellious" Yang Ki of the Liver, Gall Bladder, and Stomach, is due to Kidney Yin depletion in the early months. Treat it by first giving pressure down the Bladder Channel with folded forefinger and thumb (as shown), with your partner in the side position.

Exercises for pregnancy

Yoga classes for expectant mothers are sometimes available, but regular swimming is a good substitute, and the exercises given in this book can all be done quite safely, observing sensible limits.

Cautions:

Observe the cautions given on page 4 in this book concerning strong pressure on the Gall Bladder Channel at the top of the shoulders, and points LI 4 and Sp 6. Also avoid all the Yin Channels on the inside of the lower legs, if you are worried about the possibility of miscarriage in the early months. Other than this shiatsu is safe during pregnancy.

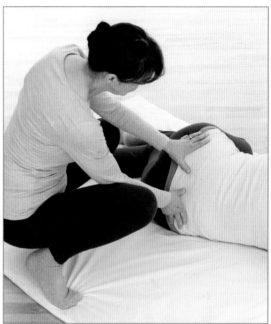

Treatment to relieve backache, haemorrhoids, and varicose veins

One of the most common complaints in the late stages of pregnancy is lower backache and tired, heavy legs. The baby's weight puts strain on the mother's spine and a downward pressure on the pelvis. Haemorrhoids and varicose veins are the more severe manifestations of circulation impeded in this way. As with other conditions, all these symptoms can be helped by working on the Bladder Channel. Begin on the back and continue all the way down the legs, first palming, then thumbing. Lean in from behind as shown.

Thumbing the sacral points for labour

Shiatsu in labour can hasten and strengthen contractions and reduce pain. It can even bring on a delayed labour and save the need for artificial induction.

In giving shiatsu you should listen to your partner's needs, but generally your work at this stage should be strong — matching any pain when it occurs. All the forbidden points now become points of choice. Strong shiatsu on the shoulders often helps to start things off. Strong thumb pressure on the sacrum is often good when pains are bad. Try LI 4, Bl 60, and Sp 6, and give pressure to tender points on the ear.

SHIATSU IN THE SITTING POSITION

You can practise shiatsu in any situation: it needs no preparation, only your versatility. Shiatsu in the sitting position is a useful means of treating people in everyday situations. But it is more than that. Elderly or disabled people may not be able to lie down easily; people suffering from asthma are often more comfortable sitting up, and it is a positive advantage to treat neck and shoulder pains or spasms in the upright position.

The major challenge of working on people in the sitting position is to provide them with support from your body while you work. Bring your leaning support into play. The routine that follows serves as basic practice, but soon you will be able to improvise and work in your own way.

Beginning the routine

If your partner is able to sit comfortably on the floor, then this is the best place to work. Ask them to kneel or sit cross-legged and offer a cushion to make either position easier. Kneeling or sitting cross-legged for 15 or 20 minutes can be difficult if you are unused to it. Encourage your partner to move if they become cramped or numb. Adapt your work to a chair or stool if that seems best.

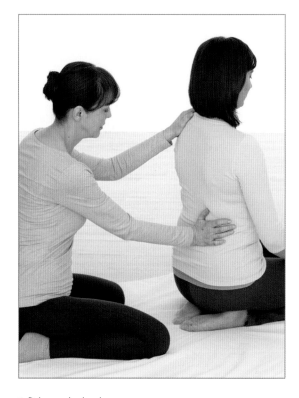

1. Palming the back

Begin by holding your partner's shoulder with your support hand and palm down the spine from between the shoulders to the sacro-lumbar region. This allows you to feel your partner's condition, especially their breathing and any stiffness in the spine. Relax your elbows and keep the pressure of your two hands equal and balanced.

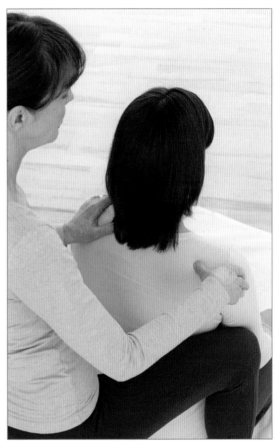

2. Leaning on the shoulders

Then move closer to support your partner's back as you give elbow pressure across your partner's shoulders starting from the corner of the neck.

3. Thumbing the shoulder Channels

Give thumb pressure along the three shoulder Channels: the Gall Bladder Channel along the top; the Triple Burner Channel just behind the muscle; and the Small Intestine Channel over the ridge of the shoulder blade. Adjust your position as you work. If you sit back to keep right-angled pressure over the shoulder blade area, try using your raised knee to support your other arm, or your partner's back directly.

Working on the Bladder and Gall Bladder Channels to clear the head

In acute illness the Yang Channels are called into play. Reacting to external influences, Yang Ki produces strong and unpleasant symptoms in the head where the Channels meet. Colds and sinus troubles, hayfever, headaches, and hangovers, as well as earache, and pain or inflammation of the eyes are common.

Treat the Bladder and Gall Bladder Channels, which run from the eye region over the top of the head (see steps 4–7, opposite and overleaf). Their courses and connecting links make them very effective in dispersing blockages, clearing the senses, and eliminating invasive climatic influences. Balance this local work with shiatsu on the back and limbs (see pp. 180–83).

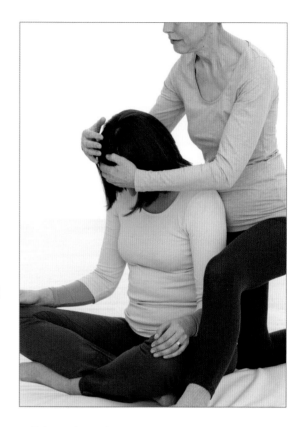

4. Relaxing the neck

Begin work on the head with this effective loosening technique for the neck. Move close and support your partner with your thigh or hip. Let your partner rest their head forward on to your overlapping palms. Keep your elbows on their shoulders and give them time to accept your support. Then raise the head a little and slide the hand touching the forehead out, allowing the head to drop a very short distance on to your other hand. Catch them securely and repeat a few times. Encourage your partner to give up control.

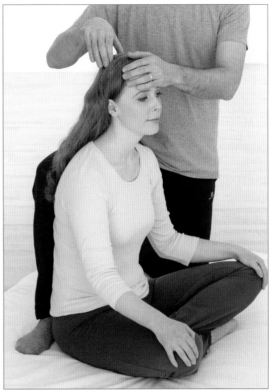

5. Finger pressure on Bladder and Gall Bladder Channels

After relaxing the neck, bring your partner's head upright and lean forward a little to support the head gently with your body. Now use your curled forefingers or middle fingers to give pressure along the Bladder, then the Gall Bladder Channels, from the eyebrows to the top of the head, as shown. Don't press. Rely on the natural weight of your arms.

6. Bladder and Gall Bladder Channels from the side position

Move to the side, raise your knee to support your partner's back with your thigh, support the forehead with one hand, and continue to give pressure with the extended thumb and forefinger of the other. Work on the Bladder and Gall Bladder Channels over the back of the head.

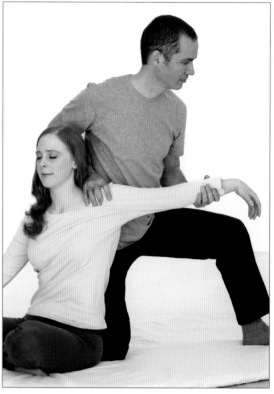

7. Rotating the head

Move your thumb and forefinger into the hollows at the base of the skull. Rotate the head gently with your support hand. Your thumb acts as a fulcrum at the base of the skull.

8. Rotating the shoulder

Before you give shiatsu down the arm, rotate the arm at the shoulder to loosen the joints and help your partner relax. Move your supporting hand to grasp the shoulder of the arm that you are working with. For ease of control hold the arm just above or below the elbow and rotate it in widening circles a few times, forward, up, back, and down. Use your whole body, not just your arm muscles, to make the movements. Move out of your own way as you pull back. Go carefully through any stiff points. If you feel your partner helping or resisting, remind them to relax.

9. Shiatsu on the arm Channels

After a few full rotations bring your partner's arm to rest on your raised thigh, a restful position for you to use. Work down the arm using the palm, thumb, or elbow (see above). The Large Intestine (see p. 90) and Triple Burner (see p. 125) are the most accessible Channels.

10. Thumb and forefinger pressure down the back

Place your arm across the front, supporting your partner's shoulders with your elbow and fingers. Take care to give your partner breathing space, and avoid contact with the neck and throat. Use the thumb and folded forefinger of your other hand to give pressure down each side of the spine. Work from the base of the neck toward the lumbar region. This technique gently opens the chest, stimulates the breath, and relaxes the whole back and spine.

11. Preparing for the full back stretch

To prepare for the next technique, a dynamic back stretch (see p. 183), stand behind your partner and clasp their hands firmly by the sides of the wrists, in the cleft between the bones (see right). A firm grip here prevents stretching the skin when you lift.

Make a number of preliminary rotations, carrying the arms up, back, and down again, reminding your partner to relax their shoulders and elbows.

Wrist clasp

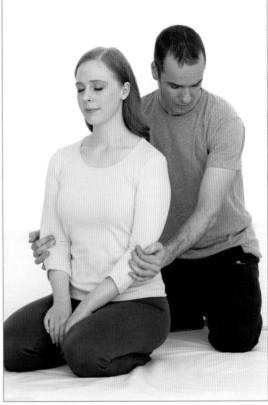

12. The full back stretch

After one or two loosening rotations, lift your partner's arms up. Find a suitable angle to support the back against your knee and thigh by adjusting the position of your front foot, then ask your partner to relax backward, pause for a moment and suggest they inhale then exhale. On the outward breath stretch your partner up and back, using your knee as a fulcrum and transferring your weight to your back foot. Release the arms, circle them round, adjust your knee up or down a little, and repeat the rotations once or twice.

13. Squeezing and releasing the shoulders and arms

Replace your partner's arms on their lap after the final stretch and, kneeling down behind, place your hands on their shoulders for a moment. Let them settle. Then squeeze and release the shoulder muscles several times. Continue this grip-release action across the shoulders and then on down the arms in quick succession. Then "brush" down the shoulders and arms to smooth the Ki.

Finishing the routine

It is, as always, best to finish the routine as you began. Sit back slightly, support one shoulder and give quiet contact in one or two places down your partner's spine with your open palm. Then they will feel settled. Let them know that you have finished. In shiatsu, the question of when and how to finish is as important to practise as the quality of attention in our first touch.

Shiatsu means relationship –
more than just "finger pressure".
Having hands we reach out to receive
and we extend ourselves in work.
Being heavy we need something to lean on,
the Earth lends us her body for support.
In shiatsu our partners lend their body for support.
Then, resting and strong,
we can offer our hand in help.
Breathing Heaven's Spirit,
two people,
really one.

INDEX

BIBLIOGRAPHY

Beijing, Shanghai, & Nanjing Colleges of Traditional Medicine with The Acupuncture Inst. of the Academy of Traditional Chinese Medicine, Essentials of Chinese Acupuncture, Foreign Languages Press (China), 1980

Kaptchuk, Ted J., Chinese Medicine: The Web that has no Weaver, Century Hutchinson (UK), Congdon and Weed Inc. (US), 1983

Lao Tzu Tao Teh Ching (Lau D. C. English trans), Penguin (UK), 1963. (Feng, Gia-Fu & Jane English trans), Random House (US), 1972

Lo, Inn, Amacker, Foe, The Essence of Tai Chi Ch'uan, North Atlantic Press (US), 1979

Maciocia, Giovanni, Foundations of Chinese Medicine, Churchill Livingstone (UK and US), 1989

Masunaga, Shizuto with Wataru Ohashi, Zen Shiatsu, Japan Publications, 1977

Matsumoto, K. and S. Birch, Five Elements and Ten Stems, Paradigm Publications (US), 1983

Shangdong Medical College & Shangdong College of Traditional Chinese Medicine, Anatomical Atlas of Chinese Acupuncture Points, Shangdong Science and Technology Press (China), 1982

Shanghai College of Traditional Medicine (O'Connor, J. & D. Bensky, trans and ed) Acupuncture: A Comprehensive Text, Eastland Press (US), 1981

Veith, Ilza (trans), The Yellow Emperor's Classic of International Medicine, University of California Press (US), 1972

Wilhelm, R. (trans), The I Ching or Book of Changes, (Baynes, C. F. English rendition), Routledge Kegan Paul Ltd (UK), 1950

Wu, Zhang Ming & Sun Xingyuan, Chinese Qi Gong Therapy, Shangdong Science and Technology Press (China), 1985

FURTHER READING

Beresford-Cooke, Carola, *Shiatsu Theory and Practice*, Churchill Livingstone (UK), 2011

Chuen, Lam Kam, *The Way of Energy*, Gaia Books (UK), Simon & Schuster (US & Australia), 1991

Flaws, Bob and Honora Wolfe, *Prince Wen Hui's Cook: Chinese Dietary Therapy*, Paradigm Publications (US), 1983

Jarmey, Chris and John Timdall, *Acupressure for Common Ailments*, Gaia Books (UK), Simon & Schuster (US), Angus & Robertson (Australia), 1991

Kishi, Akinobu and Alice Whieldon Sei-ki, *Life in Resonance – The Secret Art of Shiatsu*, Singing Dragon (UK and US), 2011

Langre, Jacques de, *Do-in2: The Ancient Art of Rejuvenation Through Self-Massage*, Happiness Press (US), 1981

Scott, Julian, *Natural Medicine for Children*, Unwin Hyman (UK & Australia), Avon Books (US), 1990

Seem, Mark, *Bodymind Energetics: Towards a Dynamic Model of Health*, Thorsons (UK), 1987

RESOURCES

For further study and training in shiatsu, contact the following:

UK

The Shiatsu Society (UK)
PO Box 4580
Rugby CV21 9BL
www.shiatsusociety.org
E-mail:admin@shiatsusociety.org
Tel: 0845 130 4560

The Shiatsu College
Various branches throughout the UK
www.shiatsucollege.co.uk

Australia

Australian Natural Therapists Association
Suite 1, 2nd Floor
468–472 George Street
(PO Box A964)
Sydney NSW 2000
www.australiannaturaltherapistsassociation.com.au

USA

American Organization for Bodywork Therapy of Asia
1010 Haddonfield–Berlin Road, Suite 408
Voorhees, NJ 08043-3514
www.aobta.org
Tel: (856) 782-1616

ACKNOWLEDGEMENTS

"Recognize, the grandfathers have said, that nothing unnatural exists. And that when man knows the truth, the whole truth, he gives name to that which he once called mystery; and that when a man needs to know something, a teacher appears."

LAKOTAH INDIAN HANTA YO:
CLEAR THE WAY
RUTH HILL

AUTHOR'S ACKNOWLEDGEMENTS

Many teachers have helped me on my way and for their presence and guidance I feel always deeply grateful. I would like to thank first of all Bill Tara, who set my feet (and hands) on the shiatsu path, Gideon Ron, who nudged me forward, and Wataru Ohashi for his inspiring early seminars in London. I am particularly indebted to Giovanni Maciocia, who taught me acupuncture and who first laid out clearly for me the disciplines and wonders of Chinese Medicine. Special thanks also to Michael Rose for his insightful and very individual shiatsu teaching.

I am grateful to have studied Masunaga's shiatsu style with Pauline Sasaki (1946–2010), who graciously responded to the call when first invited to England and subsequently inspired a whole generation of European shiatsu students with her developments of the work.

My deepest appreciation and gratitude go to Akinobu Kishi (1949–2012), my most beloved, constant, and challenging teacher, whose great gift was to show, through the practice of Seiki, how to set aside all formal knowledge, surrender to feeling, and trust in life, in nature and in the mystery of the Tao, the only thing that endures.

I would also like to remember Helena Thomas, my first yoga teacher, whose Iyengar Institute in Brighton was a light in darkness, and Kieth and Linda Codling for their guidance and healing sanctuary. Thanks also to Simon Wyard, my first Taiji teacher, Fabian Maman who opened the Daoyin path for me and especially to the late Dr Shen Hongxun for his deep wisdom and original teaching of Daoyin Qigong.

This is an opportunity to record my appreciation for the ongoing work of The Shiatsu Society in Britain and more particularly to acknowledge, with heartfelt thanks, my friends and colleagues in The Shiatsu College whose warmth and comradeship on this long journey I have been privileged to share. Thanks also to all my students, from whom I continue to learn.

I would like to record my continuing gratitude to Eleanor Lines, my editor, and Dave Thorp, designer at Gaia Books, for their dedicated professionalism and support during the work on the original edition of this book. Thanks also to Linda Sontag and those at Aardvark Editorial for their work on the revised 2004 edition. For this edition special thanks go to the editors (Liz Dean, Katy Denny, Alex Stetter) and to the design and photography team (Penny Stock, Abigail Read, Ruth Jenkinson). Thanks, finally, to all those who have modelled for this project and especially to my friend Paula Cox, whose drawings eloquently enhance the interpretation of some major themes.

Personal thanks go to my family and friends for the love, understanding and support on which I do rely, especially to my constant daughters, Tamlin and Georgina, and to my partner, Marina, always by my side.

PICTURE ACKNOWLEDGEMENTS

Bridgeman Art Library: © British Library Board. All Rights
Reserved 55; Fitzwilliam Museum, University of Cambridge,
UK 147; © FuZhai Archive 155; Leeds Museums and
Galleries (Leeds Art Gallery) U.K. 150; Private Collection 13,
25; Victoria and Albert Museum, London, UK 149.
Getty Images: 41; De Agostini 153.
Octopus Publishing Group: Adrian Pope 156. Thinkstock
Hemera: 14 below.

PUBLISHER'S ACKNOWLEDGEMENTS

Gaia Books would like to thank Alvin Attry, Edwina
Cheng, Georgie Deverell, Alice Fixsen, Kathy Hulme,
Tanya Latimore, Paul Lundberg, Uli Packer, Pam Thorpe,
Greg Tull, Maki Uegaki, Lee Willocks and Matt Woods
for modelling.

Commissioning Editor: Liz Dean
Editors: Katy Denny, Alex Stetter
Art Directors: Jonathan Christie, Penny Stock
Designer: Penny Stock
Photographer: Ruth Jenkinson
Illustrators: Abigail Read, Paula Cox (pp. 68, 78, 98, 122)
Production Controller: Allison Gonsalves